Toxic Young Adulthood

This book is for those interested in providing psychotherapy and counselling for young adults, and those who wish to bring a therapeutic sensibility to working with this client group.

Two main questions are addressed: What are the implications of providing a therapeutic ethos for young adults; and what, if any, additional training might be required for psychotherapists and counsellors working with this client group? In so doing this book explores what has too long been seen, at least for childhood, to be an urgent need for a therapeutic ethos. Such an ethos is to bring both therapeutic and educational sensibilities to bear on preventative and curative approaches to issues of young adults' well-being.

The chapters in this book, except one, were originally published in the *European Journal of Psychotherapy & Counselling*.

Del Loewenthal is an emeritus professor of Psychotherapy and Counselling at the University of Roehampton, UK, and is the chair of the Southern Association for Psychotherapy and Counselling (SAFPAC), London, UK. He is an existential-analytic psychotherapist, and a chartered psychologist, with a particular interest in phenomenology. His books include *Existential Psychotherapy and Counselling after Postmodernism* (Routledge 2017). www.delloewenthal.com; www.safpac.co.uk

Toxic Young Adulthood

Therapy and Therapeutic Ethos

Edited by
Del Loewenthal

Routledge
Taylor & Francis Group

LONDON AND NEW YORK

First published 2023
by Routledge
4 Park Square, Milton Park, Abingdon, Oxon, OX14 4RN

and by Routledge
605 Third Avenue, New York, NY 10158

Routledge is an imprint of the Taylor & Francis Group, an informa business

Introduction and Chapter 8 © 2023 Del Loewenthal
Chapters 1-7 © 2023 Taylor & Francis

British Library Cataloguing-in-Publication Data
A catalogue record for this book is available from the British Library

ISBN13: 978-1-032-19605-3 (hbk)
ISBN13: 978-1-032-19606-0 (pbk)
ISBN13: 978-1-003-26000-4 (ebk)

DOI: 10.4324/9781003260004

Typeset in Minion Pro
by codeMantra

Publisher's Note
The publisher accepts responsibility for any inconsistencies that may have arisen during the conversion of this book from journal articles to book chapters, namely the inclusion of journal terminology.

Disclaimer
Every effort has been made to contact copyright holders for their permission to reprint material in this book. The publishers would be grateful to hear from any copyright holder who is not here acknowledged and will undertake to rectify any errors or omissions in future editions of this book.

Contents

Citation Information

The following chapters were originally published in the *European Journal of Psychotherapy & Counselling*, volume 22, issue 3–4 (2020). When citing this material, please use the original page numbering for each article, as follows:

Chapter 1
The time it takes; How do we understand personal growth in an age of instant solutions?
Rowan Williams
European Journal of Psychotherapy and Counselling, volume 22, issue 3–4 (2020) pp. 208–217

Chapter 2
Training for counselling young people – What is added by a child and adolescent specialism?
Susan Kegerreis
European Journal of Psychotherapy and Counselling, volume 22, issue 3–4 (2020) pp. 173–191

Chapter 3
The narratives of parental alienation
Sally Parsloe
European Journal of Psychotherapy and Counselling, volume 22, issue 3–4 (2020) pp. 192–207

Chapter 4
What differend do you make? An imaginary phenomenology of working with a young adult
Tony McSherry
European Journal of Psychotherapy and Counselling, volume 22, issue 3–4 (2020) pp. 218–232

Chapter 5

Finishing school, fishing and flourishing: Appetite, engagement and compliance in Daoism, Existentialism and Psychoanalysis
Onel Brooks
European Journal of Psychotherapy and Counselling, volume 22, issue 3–4 (2020) pp. 233–254

Chapter 6

The golden cage
Bice Benvenuto
European Journal of Psychotherapy and Counselling, volume 22, issue 3–4 (2020) pp. 255–267

Chapter 7

How might a therapeutic ethos serve young adults? – A commentary on the theme issue
Richard House
European Journal of Psychotherapy and Counselling, volume 22, issue 3–4 (2020) pp. 268–283

For any permission-related enquiries please visit:
http://www.tandfonline.com/page/help/permissions

Notes on Contributors

Bice Benvenuto is a psychoanalyst practising in London, a founding member of the *Centre for Freudian Analysis and Research*, the director of *Associazione Dolto* in Rome and a founder of the Maison Verte-UK in London. For many years she has been a visiting professor at the *New School of Social Research* (NY) and *Florida Atlantic* University, and has lectured extensively in the UK and abroad on psychoanalysis, feminine sexuality, child analysis and literature.

Onel Brooks is particularly interested in philosophy and psychoanalysis. He is a member of the core teaching team of SAFPAC (www.safpac.co.uk); a senior lecturer in Psychotherapy, Counselling and Counselling Psychology in Psychology Department at Roehampton University, UK; and BACP-accredited and UKCP-registered as a psychoanalytic psychotherapist and as an existential analytic psychotherapist.

Richard House is a chartered psychologist, a childhood campaigner, and a 'former' lots of things –including the university lecturer in Psychology and Education Studies, a counsellor-therapist, and a Steiner Kindergarten leader and trained Steiner class teacher. Author or (co-) editor of 14 books, Richard's best-selling book *Too Much, Too Soon? Early Learning and the Erosion of Childhood* was published in 2011; and his latest book is *Pushing back to Ofsted* (2020). Richard is currently a full-time left-green activist in Gloucestershire.

Susan Kegerreis is a senior lecturer in the Department of Psychosocial and Psychoanalytic Studies at the University of Essex, UK. Having trained in both child and adolescent psychotherapy and adult psychotherapy she has practised in health, education and community settings, as well as in private practice. She has led or taught on a range of psychotherapy and counselling trainings.

Del Loewenthal is an emeritus professor of Psychotherapy and Counselling at the University of Roehampton, UK, and is the chair of the Southern Association for Psychotherapy and Counselling (SAFPAC), London, UK. He is an existential-analytic psychotherapist, and a chartered psychologist, with a particular interest in phenomenology. His books include *Existential Psychotherapy and Counselling after Postmodernism* (Routledge 2017).

Tony McSherry is an existential-analytical psychotherapist working in private practice in Liverpool.

Sally Parsloe completed an MSc in Counselling and Psychotherapy at Roehampton University, UK. She has worked in the NHS and as a therapist within a Family Mediation organisation in London. She now has a private practice in London as a psychotherapist and as a couples counsellor. She is a member of the Southern Association of Psychotherapists and Counsellors (SAFPAC) and is the chair of the SAFPAC Ethics Committee. She is also a member of the Critical Psychotherapy Network.

Rowan Williams taught theology in Cambridge and Oxford before becoming Bishop of Monmouth in Wales (1992–2002) and later Archbishop of Canterbury (2002–2012). From 2013 to 2020 he was Master of Magdalene College, Cambridge. He now lives in Wales. He is the author of several books on theology and spirituality.

Introduction – toxic young adulthood: therapy and therapeutic ethos

Del Loewenthal

At the time of writing, we do not know the full effects of the coronavirus on young adults with it interrupting their education, social development and job prospects. Yet we do know that tragically they will both be paying, in many ways, and that the pre-existing roots of young people's malaise has already for too long been deep rooted.

This book is both for those interested in providing psychotherapy and counselling for young adults, and those who wish to bring a therapeutic sensibility to working with this client group. Two main questions are addressed: What are the implications of providing a therapeutic ethos for young adults; and what, if any, additional training might be required for psychotherapists and counsellors working with this client group?

In so doing we explore what has too long been seen, at least for childhood (see, for example, House & Loewenthal 2009), to be an urgent need for a therapeutic ethos and as with climate change may be beyond the point of no return. Such an ethos could bring both therapeutic and educational sensibilities to bear on the issue of young adults' well-being. This is considered essential, if truly effective and appropriate policy responses to the current malaise, as witnessed by a steady stream of research reports, are to be fashioned.

So is modern society really bad for young adults? Furthermore, is much of psychotherapy and counselling of adults often working with what was their young adults' (and childhood) experiences? If the answer to either of these questions is 'yes' then is there a way to minimise young adults' detrimental experiences so they can have better lives and need less therapy as adults? Indeed, shouldn't one of the aims of our society be to reduce the need for psychological therapies and have culturally and community sanctioned means for reducing, holding and supporting young people's difficulties of living? Unfortunately, it would appear that in contrast, modern technological society is responsible for generating very particular kinds of distress that are in danger of becoming normalised.

Most of the chapters in this book arose out of the same named conference I chaired at the University of Cambridge. At that time (November 2019) there were yet again disturbing reports, this one using a meta-analysis:

> There is problematic smartphone use in approximately one in every four Children and Young People and accompanied by an increased odds of poorer mental health .. [depression; anxiety; stress; poor sleep quality; and decreased educational attainment]. [This] .. is an evolving public health concern…. Policy guidance is needed to outline harm reduction strategies.
>
> (Sohn et al. 2019)

But again, are we doing anything? Are we so thoroughly alienated that we are quite unable to perceive even our own alienation? Further, the pandemic, Brexit in the UK, austerity, commodification and commercialisation are far from helping.

Instead, following Sue Palmer's *Toxic childhood* (2006), shouldn't we now be urgently also talking about "toxic young adulthood". With such toxicity should it be, to rephrase her case: *the moral responsibility of everyone, including academics and therapists to consider how we might counter the negative side effects of such aspects as modern technological culture from young adults' well-being?*

In 2007 UNICEF reported that regarding children's wellbeing Britain was at the bottom of a league table of the 21 richest countries. UNICEF's later study in 2013 did suggest an improvement in the ranking of Britain, i.e., 16 out of 29 of the world's richest countries …. With still relative problems in Britain include high teenage pregnancy, a relatively high percentage not in employment, and the lowest percentage of young people in further education among major developed nations. But this was before the subsequent severe effects of austerity where:

> The young poor were early targets for all benefits cuts: their education maintenance allowance went – up to £30 a week for 16- to 19-year-olds from lowest-income families to keep them in education, covering travel, lunches, books and pocket money. Their families lost child tax credits, child benefit and housing benefit, and were often forced to move and move again.
>
> (Toynbee 2018)

Interestingly, which might be seen as both evidence of, and contributing to the continuing 'decline of the West', in both of UNICEF's studies the USA (which the UK seems to be moving towards) is near the bottom of both reports. The Institute of Medicine and National Research Council's *Investing in The Health and Well-Being of Young Adults* makes the case that young adults should be considered as a separate group from adolescents and older adults. They state:

> Young adulthood – ages approximately 18 to 26 – is a critical period of development with long-lasting implications for a person's economic security, health and well-being.
>
> (Institute of Medicine and National Research Council 2015)

Should we be propelling young adults' well-being onto the media agenda?

I was a signatory to the first public letter organised by Sue Palmer and Richard House entitled 'Modern life leads to more depression amongst children' published in the *Daily Telegraph* on 12th December 2006. This had some considerable success in drawing attention to what many believed to be the increasing incidence of mental health problems. It quickly turned into a news story spreading across the globe. Hypothetically, what might this letter look like now like if rather than children we spoke of young adults?

"Sir

As professionals and academics from a range of background we are increasingly concerned at the escalating incidence of young adulthood depression and their behavioural and developmental concerns. We believe this is largely due to a lack of understanding on the part of both politicians and the general public of the realities and subtitles of the development of young adults. Their brains cannot adjust to evermore rapid technological and cultural change…. They are pushed by market forces and exposed to unprecedented pressures on social media. Our society seems less interested in protecting them from physical harm but seems even more so to have lost sight of their emotional and social needs. The mental health of an unacceptable number of young adults is being unnecessarily compromised and this is almost a key factor in the rise of substance abuse, violence and self-harm amongst them. This is a socio-cultural problem to which there is no simple solution, but a possible first step would be to encourage parents and policy makers to start talking more about ways of improving young adult's wellbeing. We therefore propose as a matter of urgency the public debate being initiated on helping young adults in the 21st century and that this issue should be central to public policy making in coming decades.

Yours …."

Working therapeutically with young adults

To now turn to our second theme involving working therapeutically with young adults and in particular whether this requires specialist training.

In, for example, the United Kingdom Council for Psychotherapy if you want to advertise that you are available for child and adolescent work you have to undertake a specialist training and/ or engage in specific CPD. How important is this?

One argument for a different or additional training might be that those only trained to work with adults do not have sufficient ability to facilitate young adult 'play' in a similar, though different way to children. If this is the case then shouldn't we be concerned that the tendency towards a utilitarian instrumental mindset and 'development – obsessiveness' that can dominate modern learning unwittingly makes play into a thing – an object being manipulated by adults which, in turn, fatally compromises the essence of truly authentic playing?

Arising out of the above-mentioned Toxic Childhood letter Richard House and I both ran a conference (which included many members of the-then UK shadow cabinet) and subsequently a conference on play and playfulness (see EJPC 2008) introducing it with the following quotation which I think has implications for working therapeutically with any age group:

> Play has an essence which is completely independent of the attitude of the player. If this is not realised, then play becomes distorted *by being cultivated*, as is commonly done in both education and psychotherapeutic circles... all playing is a being played... [it] does not allow the player to behave towards it like an object... play does not point to purposes beyond itself, it celebrates itself... *Its nature is completely distorted if this is considered psychologistically as a known thing about which assertions can be made and people then set forth to cultivate.* [own emphasis]
>
> (Heaton 1978)

Surely the psychological therapies can certainly help us as a vehicle for learning again through a different kind and quality of relational experience. However, a preventative sense may be even more vital for the quality of formal and informal educational experience in general in terms of a therapeutic ethos be addressed in our wider culture.

For such concern for the soul, as is entailed in psychotherapy and education to effectively enhance our well-being, Plato's argument is that focus needs to be more on dialogue. How can we minimise being corrupted? Plato argues that virtue is a precondition for knowledge and that well-being is inaccessible to corrupt minds. But can we facilitate and enable young people to come away from what may be corrupting? Can virtue be imparted and acquired through the psychological therapies? And is there the necessary political will to impart it more generally in our society? Such approaches would be in direct contrast to those that might take our minds off anything that causes us to be anxious or depressed.

There is the further question relating to the training of psychological therapists not only with regard to specifically working with young adults but with regard to which a more explicitly psychosocial dimension might be more helpful. Further, psychotherapists 'values' could also be explored in terms of changing political, economic, social and technological contexts.

Don't we all as psychotherapists have a shared ethical responsibility to do all we can to protect young adults from more intrusively poisonous low-trust values that the audit culture at its worst represents and actively cultivates? To the extent that we fail there promises to be a too long queue at our door for years to come.

I would like to end this part of this Introduction to our book with two quotes, the first of which is also in Chapter 8. I think they indicate the need for a different thinking to that which currently and disastrously dominates if we are going to achieve any effective insight, both as therapists and as policy-makers, into what I am terming here 'toxic young adulthood'.

If we allow Plato to speak, he will suggest that a question before us is whether we will shrivel on the positivistic vine or with him, plumb again the resources of the human soul and so recover...

(Cushman 2002)

Getting hold of the difficulty *deep down* is what is hard. Because if it is grasped near the surface it simply remains the difficulty it was. It has to be pulled out by the roots: and that involves our beginning to think about these changes in a new way.... A new way of thinking is what is hard to establish.

(Ludvig Wittgenstein, quoted in Newman 1995)

I will now introduce the chapters of our book and include some comments from the peer reviewers. Chapter 1, 'The Time It Takes: How do we understand personal growth in an age of instant solutions', is by Rowan Williams. Here, Rowan explores how the increasing commodification of experience leads to a sense of pervasive loss. He argues that to create the conditions for mental health requires a cultural resistance, which needs to be nurtured as part of any strategy for improving mental health.

"This is a beautifully written paper. It flows immaculately from one convincing argument to the next, creating thus narrative consistency and continuity and an intentional correspondence between the paper's style and content."

Chapter 2, 'Training for counselling young people – what is added by a child and adolescent specialism' is by Susan Kegerreis. Susan argues, with examples, that a specialist training to work with children and adolescents provides a significantly different valuable perspective.

"A clear, engaging and timely article that illustrates the importance of specialist training for supporting young people, and beautifully illustrated with examples."

Chapter 3, Sally Parsloe's 'The Narratives of Parental Alienation', explores that one parent uses their power over a child to excommunicate the other parent. Sally considers the possible effects of this for the child's mind and emotional landscape and how therapists may help young people to make sense of such experiences.

"It's good (and interesting)."

Tony McSherry in his Chapter 4, 'Looking back with meaning: An imaginary phenomenology of working with a young adult' asks the question: 'How do we provide a safe space for a young person to speak and find their own way without imposing the co-ordinates of our own lives upon them? Tony suggests one answer '... is to be prepared to let go of our firm beliefs and ideas, without rancour, in the face of the energy and curiosity of youth'.

"This paper promotes and highlights the importance of clients 'especially young adults' in finding their own language (words) without the presence of the other. It does so by presenting an imaginary phenomenology of working with a young adult."

Chapter 5 is 'Finishing school, fishing and flourishing Appetite, engagement and compliance in Daoism, Existentialism and Psychoanalysis'. As Onel comments such writers '... emphasise vastness, complexity, ambiguity, contrasting this with our smallness, finitude, our limitedness, our tendency to conform, comply and crave certainty. In contrast to technological thinking and convictions, they favour and show a kind of indirectness, meandering, a freedom to associate and wander....'

"It was a pleasure to read this beautifully crafted and provocative paper."

Turning now to our two published respondents. The first, Chapter 6, is Bice Benvenuto who in her fascinatingly innovative 'The golden cage' argues that the key issue in the above chapters lies in the interconnection between therapeutic and social ethos. Bice suggests a connection particularly affecting young adults between the objects of immediate satisfaction such as high-tech gadgets and their solitary enjoyment with the autistic spectrum, which has become the mental paradigm. Here commodity-based and calculative modes of *non-thinking* have become the norm, which do not allow addressing a call towards the other.

Our second respondent is Richard House. His Chapter 7 is entitled: 'How might a therapeutic ethos serve young adults? – a commentary'. Within this vitally pertinent, wide-ranging response Richard significantly emphasises the importance of therapists '...*not to get in the way of* the complex developmental struggles of the troubled young adults who find their way into therapy.'

Finally in Chapter 8, 'Young adulthood, wellbeing and a therapeutic ethos: A case for therapeutic education', I argue that we first need to consider, with the help of Plato's *Therapeia*, what it might mean for our society to have an appropriate therapeutic ethos, and how we might achieve this. Only then can we consider whether current notions, such as audit, are helpful or detrimental to this purpose. In order to illustrate this, the term 'well-being' is explored and, in particular, how with appropriate therapeutic education we can provide an enabling, dynamic environment both for our children and young adults and, through them, for ourselves, which in turn potentially enables us to make a better world.

There are many people to thank for this book in addition, and thank you again for the above contributors. These include: Evrinomy Avdi, Julia Cayne, Yana Flint, Anastasios Gaitanidis, Seth Osborne, Jay Watts and David Winter. However, there is one person without whom in particular this book and this editorial would not have been possible and that is Richard House. Richard not only helped me significantly in devising the initial conference, from which this special issue developed, but also influenced me so much through our previous work on childhood and play. I would indeed like to end by again adapting something we previously wrote (House & Loewenthal 2009):

A key theme of this book is that we urgently need a therapeutic ethos in order to bring both educational and therapeutic sensibilities to bear on young adults' well-being, if truly effective and appropriate policy responses to the current malaise are to be fashioned. Not least, we must pay particular attention to young adult's experience, showing that scientific and technical developments are always secondary to the resources of the human soul, if we are to minimise the extent to which today's young adults will need therapy as adults. This will entail moving beyond narrowly mechanistic definitions of, and ways of thinking about, "well-being" and the psychological therapies. It is further very much hoped that this book is not only for psychotherapists but offers pointers the kinds of arguments that can inform what needs to rapidly become a central concern of politicians and policymakers.

References

Cushman, R. (2002). *Therapeia: Plato's Conception of Philosophy*. New Brunswick and London: Transaction Publishers.

EJPC (*European Journal of Psychotherapy & Counselling*) (2008). Special Issue on Play and Playfulness, ed. R. House & D. Loewenthal, vol. 10 (2).

Heaton, J. (1978). 'The Ontology of Play.' In: B. Curtis and W. Mays (Eds) *Phenomenology and Education*. London: Methuen, pp. 119–130.

House, R. and Loewenthal, D. (2009). *Childhood, Wellbeing and a Therapeutic Ethos.* London: Karnac.

Institute of Medicine and National Research Council (2015). *Investing in the Health and Well-Being of Young Adults.* Washington, DC: The National Academies Press. https://doi.org/10.17226/18869

Newman, S. (1995). *Philosophy and Teacher Education.* London: Routledge Revivals.

Palmer, S. (2006). *Toxic Childhood.* London: Orion.

Sohn, S., Rees, P., Wildridge, B. et al. (2019). 'Prevalence of Problematic Smartphone Usage and Associated Mental Health Outcomes Amongst Children and Young People: A Systematic Review, Meta-Analysis and GRADE of the Evidence.' *BMC Psychiatry*, 19, 356.

Toynbee, P. (2018). 'Cut Youth Services and Violent Crime Will Rise – Is That Really So Hard to See?' *The Guardian*, 5th April 2018.

UNICEF (2007). *Child Poverty in Perspective: An Overview of Child Wellbeing in Rich Countries.* Innocenti Report Card 7, UNICEF Innocenti Research Centre, Florence.

The time it takes; How do we understand personal growth in an age of instant solutions?

Rowan Williams

ABSTRACT

One source of the mental health challenges facing contemporary people, especially younger people, is the increasing commodification of experience: phases of life, human encounters and so on, which were once part of a connected narrative are seen as items to be purchased/acquired/accumulated by a curiously contentless desiring ego. But the effect of this is a sense of pervasive loss – characterised as loss of rhythm, narrative and future. There is a loss of connection with the processes and agencies of the natural world, a loss of a continuous narrative of the self and a loss of a manageable or desirable future (individual and social). Creating the conditions for mental health (not simply providing ambulance services) requires cultural resistance in all these areas; it is important to identify and nurture signs of such resistance as part of any strategy for improving mental health.

Die Zeit, die es braucht; Wie verstehen wir persönliches Wachstum im Zeitalter sofortiger Lösungen

ABSTRAKT

Eine Quelle für die psychischen Gesundheitsprobleme, mit denen zeitgenössische Menschen, insbesondere jüngere Menschen, konfrontiert sind, ist die zunehmende Vermarktung von Erfahrungen: Lebensphasen, menschliche Begegnungen usw., die einst Teil einer zusammenhängenden Erzählung waren, werden als zu kaufende/zu erwerbende Gegenstände angesehen. Angesammelt durch ein merkwürdig inhaltsloses Wunsch-Ego. Der Effekt davon ist jedoch ein Gefühl des allgegenwärtigen Verlusts - gekennzeichnet als Verlust von Rhythmus, Erzählung und Zukunft. Es gibt einen Verlust der Verbindung zu den Prozessen und Agenturen der natürlichen Welt, einen Verlust einer kontinuierlichen Selbsterzählung und einen Verlust einer überschaubaren oder wünschenswerten Zukunft (individuell und sozial). Die Schaffung der Bedingungen für die psychische Gesundheit (nicht nur die Bereitstellung von Krankenwagen) erfordert kulturellen Widerstand in all diesen Bereichen. Es ist wichtig, Anzeichen eines solchen Widerstands als Teil einer Strategie zur Verbesserung der psychischen Gesundheit zu identifizieren und zu fördern

El tiempo que se requiere; ¿Cómo entendemos el crecimiento personal en una era de soluciones instantáneas

RESUMEN

Una fuente de los desafíos de salud mental a los que se enfrentan las personas contemporáneas, especialmente las personas más jóvenes, es la creciente mercantilización de la experiencia: fases de la vida, encuentros humanos, etc., que alguna vez fueron parte de una narrativa conectada y que son vistos como elementos para ser comprados/adquiridos/acumulados por un ego curiosamente sin contenido. Pero el efecto de esto es una sensación de pérdida generalizada, caracterizada como pérdida de ritmo, historia y futuro. Hay una pérdida de conexión con los procesos y factores del mundo natural, una pérdida de una narrativa continua del yo y una pérdida de un futuro manejable o deseable (individual y social). La creación de las condiciones para la salud mental (no sólo la prestación de servicios de ambulancia) requiere resistencia cultural en todas estas áreas; es importante identificar y nutrir los signos de dicha resistencia como parte de cualquier estrategia para mejorar la salud mental.

Il tempo che occorre; Come comprendere la crescita personale in un'era di soluzioni istantanee

ASTRATTO

Una sfida per la salute mentale che deve essere affrontata dalle persone del nosro tempo, in particolare i giovani, è la crescente mercificazione dell'esperienza: fasi della vita, incontri umani e così via, che un tempo facevano parte di una narrativa sono visti come oggetti da acquistare/acquisire/accumulato da un ego desideroso curiosamente privo di contenuto. Ma l'effetto di questo è un senso di perdita pervasiva - caratterizzato come perdita di ritmo, narrativa e futuro. C'è una perdita di connessione con i processi e le agenzie del mondo naturale, una perdita di una narrazione continua di sé e una perdita di un futuro gestibile o desiderabile (individuale e sociale). Creare le condizioni per la salute mentale (non semplicemente fornire servizi di ambulanza) richiede resistenza culturale in tutte queste aree; è importante identificare e alimentare i segni di tale resistenza come parte di qualsiasi strategia per migliorare la salute mentale.

Le temps nécessaire; comprendre le développement personnel à une époque de solutions instantanées

En matière de santé mentale, un des défis auquel les gens d'aujourd'hui sont confrontés, et plus particulièrement les jeunes, est la tendance à la hausse de la marchandisation de l'expérience: les phases de la vie, les rencontres humaines et ainsi de suite, qui constituaient autrefois les éléments d'un récit connecté sont maintenant considérées comme des objets à acheter/se procurer/accumuler par un ego désirant mais curieusement sans contenu. Le résultat est un sentiment de perte omniprésent – caractérisé par une perte de rythme, de narratif et de futur. Il y a une perte de connexion avec les processus et le pouvoir de la nature, une perte de narratif continu de soi et une perte d'un futur gérable ou désirable (individuellement et socialement). Créer les conditions pour la santé mentale (et pas seulement octroyer plus de moyens aux services ambulanciers) nécessite une résistance culturelle dans tous ces domaines; il est important d'identifier et de cultiver les signes d'une telle résistance comme faisant partis de toutes stratégies visant à améliorer la santé mentale.

Ο χρόνος που χρειάζεται. Πώς αντιλαμβανόμαστε την προσωπική ανάπτυξη σε μια εποχή στιγμιαίων λύσεων

ΠΕΡΊΛΗΨΗ
Μια πηγή πρόκλησης στη ψυχική υγεία των σύγχρονων ανθρώπων, ιδίως των νεότερων, αφορά την αυξανόμενη εμπορευματοποίηση των εμπειριών: οι φάσεις της ζωής, οι ανθρώπινες συναναστροφές και ούτω καθεξής, που κάποτε ήταν μέρος μιας συνδεδεμένης αφήγησης. Πλέον θεωρούνται αντικείμενα που πρέπει να αγοραστούν/αποκτηθούν/συσσωρευτούν από ένα άδειο εγώ που έχει περιέργεια και επιδιώκει. Το αποτέλεσμα όμως, είναι μια αίσθηση διάχυτης απώλειας - που χαρακτηρίζεται ως απώλεια ρυθμού, αφήγησης και μέλλοντος. Υπάρχει απώλεια σύνδεσης με τις διαδικασίες και τις υπηρεσίες του φυσικού κόσμου, απώλεια μιας ενιαίας αφήγησης του εαυτού και απώλεια ενός διαχειρίσιμου ή επιθυμητού μέλλοντος (ατομικό και κοινωνικό). Η δημιουργία συνθηκών ψυχικής υγείας (όχι απλώς η παροχή πυροσβεστικών λύσεων) απαιτεί πολιτιστική αντίσταση σε όλους αυτούς τους τομείς. Είναι σημαντικό να εντοπίσουμε και να καλλιεργήσουμε σημάδια τέτοιας αντίστασης ως μέρος οποιασδήποτε στρατηγικής για τη βελτίωση της ψυχικής υγείας.

SCHLÜSSELWÖRTER Körperlichkeit; Ware; Umweltkrise; Erzählung

PALABRAS CLAVE corpaje; mercantilización; crisis ambiental; narrativa

PAROLE CHIAVE corporeità; mercificazione; crisi ambientale; narrativa

MOTS-CLÉS corporéité; marchandisation; crise environnementale; narrative

ΛΈΞΕΙΣ ΚΛΕΙΔΙΆ σωματικότητα; εμπορευματοποίηση; περιβαλλοντική κρίση; αφήγηση

It's not difficult, in reflecting on mental health (particularly young people's mental health) these days, to be struck by the pervasive phenomenon of the *consumerising* of human experience. More and more aspects of our lives are being reduced, explicitly or implicitly, to the level of commodities. Michael Sandel's important book, *What Money Can't Buy* (2013) did an impressive job of tracing this process of commodifying – from people paying others to stand and queue on their behalf to the bizarre practice of businesses taking out insurance on (not for) their employees to make sure of benefiting from any misfortune that happens to them. Increasingly, we are trading in the lives of others – trading time, convenience, well-being, as though these things were bits of transferable property. And the way in which we often approach human rights these days is not much help, as these too are regularly spoken of as though they were possessions, handed over to us at birth like old-fashioned Premium Bonds to be cashed when we want.

It makes rather depressing sense of the interest our institutions currently take in the quality of our experience of their work: have we had a good experience in the shop, the hospital, the school or university? Would we recommend it to other consumers? Questions about the 'student experience' in higher education institutions are a source of abiding anxiety to those who run those institutions; and the pressure on the consumer is constantly to check that you are having the best possible such experience – which involves anxious checking of our own feelings and comparing them with those of others. Somewhere in the ether there is a maximally positive experience that we should all be able to access; not a good recipe for limiting insecurity. A whole range of relationships that once had their own vocabulary and criteria are being re-imagined in these terms of producer and consumer. Student, traveller, legal client or medical patient, all are encouraged to meet on the common ground of being customers, directly or indirectly purchasing something that can succeed or fail to count as a good experience – an attitude that subtly moves us further away from asking whether a process is actually doing its job, producing a lasting outcome, whether or not we have felt it positively. Pointing this out is by no means to suggest that it is better not to think about how goods are delivered: 'successful' medical procedures in the past, to take an obvious example, were quiet often delivered in ways that infantilised or demeaned patients. But there is a real risk of blurring categories here. And the popularity of feel-good slogans in politics, blotting out hard questions about long-term results, properly effective and accountable methods and candid and sustained scrutiny, shows something of the danger. We like the sense of *immediacy* that we are offered by this stress on good experience, the sense of cutting out the interfering middle layers to secure access to what we want.

Problems enough there. But if we stop and ask about some of the underlying social factors that both explain and intensify this, the outlook becomes more complex and the problems more deep-seated. I want to try and identify some of the areas in our culture that play into the commodifying mentality, so as to raise the question of how we might step back and ask about the *conditions* for mental health, not just about diagnosis and damage limitation. And I'd sum up these areas as having to do with the awareness of *rhythm* in our human experience, with the nature of the *narrative* we tell, and with what we think and imagine about our *future*, individual and collective.

The first of these is not easy to categorise simply, but it is essentially about the ways in which we find our way to a sustainable pattern of life within the limits of our bodies. One of the most extraordinary things to surface in the last few years is the marketising of techniques to help us sleep, and the widespread confusion about this rather basic aspect of our human, embodied reality. The seductive cultural myth that associates sleep with some kind of weakness or failure in energy and aggression has sunk quite deeply into the collective psyche; we are invited to wonder at, and perhaps imitate, successful people who sleep less than the average number of hours. A globalised financial market and news cycle means that local rhythms of time keeping are felt as relative, and so perhaps unimportant: the ideal is wakefulness – not in the sense in which the word is used in the spiritual traditions of east and west as a marker for self-awareness, but as an undying vigilance around our performance and our control of the environment. As such, it is connected with the erosion of formalised or ritualised times for eating, both in house-holds and in the round of working life. The rhythms of a body that requires nourishment, relative stillness, and pauses in the flow of buts consciousness are ignored. It is true that what we habitually call 'civilised' life represents to some extent a negotiation over this: we artificially prolong hours of light, for example, to give a standardised division of day and night through the year. But this has generally remained a modification of the basic rhythm rather than a denial of the underlying structure of alternating stress and slack, systole and diastole. The problem arises when this alternation slips out of view or imagination.

Some recent commentators, like the Canadian poet Jan Zwicky, have written of our situation as one in which we are, without quite knowing it, 'homesick' for the rest of creation. It's no accident that many educational establishments invest in animals for petting at times of stress in the academic year; or that successful therapeutic programmes for young offen-ders involve giving them the care of animals. If we are regularly being persuaded to ignore our own animality, it is natural enough that the lack should be felt and that it should have damaging results; and natural that some restoration of this is part of a path to the restoration of basic well-being. Connecting with living beings that work in embodied rhythms, we are reminded of our own inescapable connection with day and night, summer and winter. And this is also why one deeply disturbing element in our current global environmental crisis is the steady reduction of forms of life around us, animate and inanimate – as if the ideal situation for human beings were to be the sole species surviving on earth.

This is further complicated by our confusions over 'narrative'. It's often pointed out that we are in a social and financial climate where any idea of a normative progression through stages of human life seems increasingly remote. Most human societies until recently worked with some broad pat-tern of growth and maturation – work, settlement in long-term sexual partnership and householding, parenthood, wider responsibility in the busi-ness of a community's life, gradual withdrawal and movement towards death. Modernity has always chafed under the implied constraints of this – not without reason, given that this could indeed be a tyrannical routine, indifferent to individual hopes and gifts, and that it was generally more repressive for women than men. But whether we are thinking of prevailing patterns of employment and the emergence of the 'portfolio career'; or of the inaccessibility of secure housing (let alone actual home ownership) for so many young people; or of the prolonging of the period of sexual experiemntation and the postponement of parenting; or of the all-or-nothing character of a lot of contemporary work, with little space for either public voluntary engagement or personal leisure – all these contribute to leaving us with a fragmented sense of personal continuity and a degree of uncertainty as to whether we can see our lives as having any cumulative shape, and progression towards some sort of balance or completeness. To put it very briefly, do we have stories about how we have learned to be human? We are regularly wary of putting the question in quite such blunt terms because of a nervousness of authorities prescriptively telling us what would count as a correct answer, and a proper awareness of the place of discontinuities, stresses and disruptions in the creation of narratives, pushing back against a premature smoothing out of stories into manageable continuity. We are sensitive to the dangers of all this because we (as people who have to some extent digested both modernism and postmodernism) are aware of the seductions of narrative *power* – my power to order and make intelligible my story about myself, my power over the narrative of another subaltern voice/perspective. The challenge is how we recover a discipline of negotiating with the material reality we all share that will produce some mutually recognisable pattern of human growth and maturity without appealing to or giving houseroom to these uncritical exercises of power. How do we come to see a truthful account of shared humanity not in terms of the ideological triumph of one party's narrative but as a carefully evolved grammar of recognition between diverse agents and cultures?

The point needs making again that addressing the deficit of contemporary imagination is not to idealise some lost golden age of fixed roles and foreordained careers; simply to note that our economic culture – determined to the point of obsession to treat us as if we lived in a series of moments of timeless consumer choice – is unfriendly to the idea that the taking of time is essential to handling the most significant questions of how we come to understand our value and our values. The consumer model is not one that gives much help in growing into tested skills and habits; and the algorithms that dictate advertising practice simply calculate regularities in moments of choice, not the processes of learning to choose, or to discriminate in our choice. When we generally lack any clear narrative at the corporate level, the story provided by a faith or a philosophy or a national history, we are left with the formidable burden of repeatedly deciding who and what we are; creating ourselves out of our own will and instinct, again and again, rather than being able to integrate a wider narrative of human development into our own record of experience and vice versa. And this also means that we are more than ever vulnerable to the lures of pre-packaged narratives promising an identity that can be readily 'weaponised': a firmly policed and defined selfhood (individual or national) divorced from any process of learning or change.

If we finally add to this the growing sense of a future that is not guaranteed to produce any augmented well-being for us as individuals or for us as a human race, the position is even more serious. The loss of a standard narrative of human development, even if resisted, critiqued, refused, turned upside down, means that we have no default confidence that there is a place to get to in our human striving. The loss of the social and economic landmarks that assured us of something like a continuous working life means that we cannot be sure that we will be 'looked after' (what are the personal and psychological effects of the steady growth of uncertainty about the performance and calculation of pension funds over the last couple of decades?). And the unavoidable images of radical environmental degradation that are before us daily cut at the very roots of any trust in a stable natural environment. The future, in short, is not only uncertain (it has always by definition been that), but more directly menacing. It is not clear why we should exert ourselves to change, grow, understand or whatever if we cannot be sure that there is in any sense a goal that has a chance of realisation. If the future is one of advancing environmental catastrophe – even perhaps in the lifetime of the present generation – our motivation is undermined at a deep level.

All of this is really to say that the global political, economic and cultural situation we inhabit at present has very few of the elements that make for mental well-being if we think of that well-being as a capacity first to own and learn from a diverse past, recognising failure and growing through testing, and also to make continuing sense of the landscape – natural and social – that we are part of. If we are concerned to serve and nurture the mental health of a younger generation, we have to look at these broad factors as well as all the local triggers that generate suffering and confusion for individuals. It is certainly true that therapeutic intervention alone is not the answer; what needs to change is more than the individual's coping mechanisms. But it is all the more important for any therapeutic activity to keep in view these wider questions, as part of the search for what I earlier called the conditions for mental health.

Recovering and sustaining mental health has to involve, sooner or later, finding strategies of resistance, personal and collective, to the various kinds of loss or displacement we have been thinking about here. In the last twelve months, we have seen the rapid development of some very dramatic strategies in connection with the environmental crisis; and the atmosphere of both the Extinction Rebellion events and the various activities of school students drawing attention to the crisis has been one in which the focus has been not exclusively on solving a problem or averting a catastrophe, but has taken on board the large questions about lasting well-being which the current situation provokes. This is something from which we can learn. There is a real concern with discovering or rediscovering ways of living positively in closer relationship with the actual limits of bodily life, and so of looking again at rhythms and disciplines that connect us afresh. And insofar as these rhythms and disciplines challenge very deeply the reactive consumerism of our times, and restore a sense that there are dimensions of our world that can't be commodified, they address the first of the concerns outlined. Once we are clearer about the fact that the world as it is itself resists the passion to reduce it to tradeable things and possessions, once we begin to recast our relation to the rest of the material cosmos as something other than a title of ownership, we may be more ready to approach our environment with the recognition that the central modern image of a 'timeless' consumer making choices among a set of fixed commodities is a dangerous fiction. And if that begins to sink in, we may be more able to ask the question of how we see both ourselves and our world as moving in time, growing, interacting and shaping a story that has some continuity. Essentially, it's a matter of coming to see that we are being *made* as we move through our encounters and our self-determinations; not 'self-made', but shaped in our possibilities and in our understanding of ourselves by the interaction between our own freedom and intelligence and the intelligent and intelligible world we negotiate.

Educational communities need to be aware of how such processes work and to guarantee space for them to be explored. This is why any educational institution that does not make room for the life of faith and the life of imagination is not going to serve the needs of its students or staff in terms of sustainable well-being. This is not only to do with traditional and familiar forms of religious and artistic engagement – and it is certainly not a matter of simply treating these things as leisure activities that can be left to the private enterprise of students. I have in mind also initiatives like the one that has recently – tragically – been in the public eye with the murder of two of its participants in the London Bridge incident last December. The Learning Together project involves students and others in accompanying prisoners through a quite demanding programme of seminars and study, designed to make prisoners and volunteers genuinely participants together in a learning process. It means for all those involved some hard questions about the story that has brought them where they are; and it presents the educational process as something dramatically other than a mere 'knowledge transfer'. It requires patience and attention and a willingness to manage the resistance, internal and external, to learning that is in different ways shared by all involved. Insofar as it is about a process aiming at a change in all those involved, it offers a narrative, a continuity, and a connectedness that should be the business of all educational endeavour.

Not for everyone, obviously; but it is one example of a strategy of resistance to the commodified world of late modernity, with its impatience and its love-affairs with instantaneous solutions and gratifications. If we want to nurture and promote mental health, it is essential to find such embodiments of the labour of building shared narratives and patterns of life that seek to be aligned with a larger world – the labour, we could say, of learning how to tell a story that is not simply 'ours'. The more we drift towards taking for granted that our human job is building identities, destinies and futures out of our isolated individuality, the more damage we are likely to do, to ourselves and our world. But that drift is not a matter of inevitable development (let alone 'progress'); it is something heavily supported by an economic climate in which the hunger for one kind of growth reduces us to an ensemble of disconnected desires and choices. Pushing back against it requires us to look for deeper resources that will help us identify deeper needs.

In this brief summary, my aim has been, first, to suggest a possible analysis of the malaise that we call commodification or consumerism, an analysis in terms of the way it invites us to ignore our bodies, our time-taking, and our instinctive pull towards story-telling; second, to note how our individual sense of discontinuity and the episodic character of our identity becomes especially problematic when it is experienced in the context of a deep fear and uncertainty about the future, individual and global; and third, to encourage us all to think about practices and strategies of pushing back, keeping alive the imagination of another style of human living that is less trapped in individual anxiety and the lure of 'self-creation', more open to acknowledging the time it takes to learn how to be in an actual *world*. In this project, the specific resources of faith and imagination – in their widest senses – need to be invoked: we need models of 'human excellence', lives lived with a continuity and integrity, an embodied wisdom and a sober hopefulness that we regularly seem to lack. Without such points of reference, we as a culture are not (as we sometimes fantasise) free and creative agents, but rather at the mercy of manipulative political forces, aggressive marketing, reductive myths of who and what we are. Should we wonder that this sort of acute and so often unrecognised vulnerability does little to secure any sense of well-being?

Disclosure statement

No potential conflict of interest was reported by the author(s).

References

Bringhurst, R., & Zwicky, J. (2019). *Learning to die: Wisdom in the age of climate crisis*. Univeisty of Regina Press.

Collini, S. (2017). *Speaking of univeristies*. Verso.

Farrell, C., Green, A., Knights, S., & Skeaping, W. (ed.). (2020). *This is not a drill: An extinction rebellion handbook*. Penguin/Random House.

Jackson, T. (2017). *Prosperity without growth: Foundations for the economy of tomorrow* (2nd ed.). Routledge.

Jones, L. (2020). *Losing Eden: Why our minds need the wild, 2020*. Penguin/Random House.

Sandel, M. (2013). *What money can't buy: The moral limits of markets*. Penguin/Random House.

Training for counselling young people – What is added by a child and adolescent specialism?

Susan Kegerreis

ABSTRACT

Working with older adolescents and young adults is somewhat disputed territory. Those with qualifications in work with adults can easily adapt to working with this age-group, and historically this has been the most usual route into the role. In this paper, I argue, however, that there is likely to be a difference between their approach and that of those who have had a specialist training to work with children and adolescents. Such trainings are likely to imbue in clinicians a much stronger awareness of: the developmental perspective; the power of ongoing family dynamics; the vexed trajectory into individual independence and identity formation and the particular vicissitudes of the learning experience. Experience of having also worked with younger children provides counsellors/therapists with a different appreciation of defensive constellations and a nuanced awareness of transference dynamics when the age and status differences between practitioner and client are greater. Working with younger people also requires a sophisticated understanding of organisational dynamics – which are less likely to feature in adult trainings. These elements provide a significantly different perspective on the work which therefore suggests that specialist training input is of great value. Examples are given in the paper to illustrate these ideas.

Schulung zur Beratung junger Menschen - was durch ein Kinder- und Jugendfach hinzugefügt wird

ABSTRAKT

Die Arbeit mit älteren Jugendlichen und jungen Erwachsenen ist ein umstrittenes Gebiet. Personen mit Qualifikationen in der Arbeit mit Erwachsenen können sich leicht an die Arbeit mit dieser Altersgruppe anpassen, und in der Vergangenheit war dies der üblichste Weg in die Rolle. In diesem Artikel argumentiere ich jedoch, dass es wahrscheinlich einen Unterschied zwischen ihrem Ansatz und dem derjenigen gibt, die eine spezielle Ausbildung für die Arbeit mit Kindern und Jugendlichen erhalten haben. Solche Schulungen werden den Klinikern wahrscheinlich ein viel stärkeres Bewusstsein vermitteln für: die Entwicklungsperspektive; die Kraft der anhaltenden Familiendynamik; der ärgerliche Weg in die individuelle Unabhängigkeit und Identitätsbildung und die besonderen Wechselfälle der Lernerfahrung. Die Erfahrung, auch mit jüngeren Kindern gearbeitet zu haben, bietet Beratern/ Therapeuten ein unterschiedliches Verständnis für defensive Konstellationen und ein differenziertes Bewusstsein für die Übertragungsdynamik, wenn die Alters- und Statusunterschiede zwischen Arzt und Klient größer sind. Die Arbeit mit jüngeren Menschen erfordert auch ein ausgefeiltes Verständnis der Organisationsdynamik, die in Schulungen für Erwachsene weniger wahrscheinlich ist. Diese Elemente bieten eine deutlich andere Perspektive auf die Arbeit, was darauf hindeutet, dass der Beitrag zur Fachausbildung von großem Wert ist. Beispiele zur Veranschaulichung dieser Ideen werden in dem Artikel gegeben. Ich behaupte jedoch, dass es wahrscheinlich einen Unterschied zwischen ihrem Ansatz und derjenigen gibt, die eine spezielle Ausbildung für die Arbeit mit Kindern und Jugendlichen erhalten haben. Solche Schulungen werden den Klinikern wahrscheinlich ein viel stärkeres Bewusstsein vermitteln für: die Entwicklungsperspektive; die Kraft der anhaltenden Familiendynamik; der ärgerliche Weg in die individuelle Unabhängigkeit und Identitätsbildung und die besonderen Wechselfälle der Lernerfahrung. Die Erfahrung, auch mit jüngeren Kindern gearbeitet zu haben, bietet Beratern/Therapeuten ein unterschiedliches Verständnis für defensive Konstellationen und ein differenziertes Bewusstsein für die Übertragungsdynamik, wenn die Alters- und Statusunterschiede zwischen Arzt und Klient größer sind. Die Arbeit mit jüngeren Menschen erfordert auch ein ausgefeiltes Verständnis der Organisationsdynamik, die in Schulungen für Erwachsene weniger wahrscheinlich ist. Diese Elemente bieten eine deutlich andere Perspektive auf die Arbeit, was darauf hindeutet, dass der Beitrag zur Fachausbildung von großem Wert ist. Beispiele zur Veranschaulichung dieser Ideen werden in dem Papier gegeben

Formación para el asesoramiento a los jóvenes – lo que se añade por una especialidad infantil y adolescente

RESUMEN

Trabajar con adolescentes mayores y adultos jóvenes es un territorio algo discutido. Aquellos cualificados para trabajar con adultos pueden adaptarse fácilmente a trabajar con este grupo de edad, e históricamente esta ha sido el papel más habitual. En este documento sostengo, sin embargo, que es probable que haya una diferencia entre su enfoque y el de aquellos que han tenido una formación especializada para trabajar con niños y adolescentes. Es probable que estas capacitaciones inculque en los médicos una conciencia mucho más fuerte de: la perspectiva del desarrollo; el poder de la dinámica familiar en curso; la discutida trayectoria hacia la independencia individual y la formación de la identidad y las vicisitudes particulares de la experiencia de aprendizaje. La experiencia de haber trabajado también con niños más pequeños proporciona a los consejeros/terapeutas una apreciación diferente de las constelaciones defensivas y una conciencia matizada de la dinámica de transferencia cuando las diferencias de edad y estado entre el practicante y el cliente son mayores. Trabajar con personas más jóvenes también requiere una comprensión sofisticada de las dinámicas organizativas, que son menos propensas a aparecer en los entrenamientos para adultos. Estos elementos proporcionan una perspectiva significativamente diferente sobre el trabajo, lo que sugiere que la aportación de formación especializada es de gran valor. En el documento se dan ejemplos para ilustrar estas ideas

Formazione per la consulenza ai giovani: cosa aggiunge uno specialismo infantile e adolescenziale

Lavorare con adolescenti e giovani adulti è alquanto controverso. Professionisti qualificati per il lavoro con gli adulti possono facilmente adattarsi a lavorare con questa fascia di età, e storicamente questa è stata la strada più usuale. In questo articolo sostengo, tuttavia, che esiste probabilmente una differenza tra l'approccio da loro utilizzato e quello di coloro che hanno avuto una formazione specialistica per lavorare con bambini e adolescenti. È probabile che specifici corsi di formazione trasmettano ai clinici una consapevolezza maggiore rispetto a: la prospettiva dello sviluppo; il potere delle dinamiche familiari in atto; la traiettoria nell'indipendenza individuale e nella formazione dell'identità e le particolari vicissitudini dell'esperienza di apprendimento. L'esperienza di lavoro anche con i bambini più piccoli fornisce ai consulenti/terapisti un diverso punto di vista delle costellazioni difensive e una consapevolezza delle particolari dinamiche di transfert quando le differenze di età e status tra professionista e cliente sono ampie. Lavorare con i giovani richiede anche una comprensione sofisticata delle dinamiche organizzative, che hanno meno probabilità di presentarsi nei corsi di formazione per adulti. Questi elementi offrono una prospettiva significativamente diversa circa il lavoro, il che suggerisce quindi che il contributo della formazione specialistica sia di grande valore. Nel contributo sono riportati esempi per meglio delineare queste idee.

Formation pour le soutien psychologique aux jeunes – ce qu'apporte une spécialité dans l'enfant et l'adolescent

Travailler avec des adolescents et des jeunes adultes est un territoire fort disputé. Ceux qui sont qualifiés pour travailler auprès d'adultes peuvent s'adapter facilement à ce groupe d'âge et historiquement c'est le chemin pris par ceux qui travaillent dans ce domaine. Dans cet article, je soutiens cependant qu'il est probable qu'il y ait une différence entre leur approche et celle de ceux qui ont suivi une formation spécialisée pour travailler avec les enfants et les adolescents. De telles formations sont susceptibles de donner aux cliniciens une plus grande conscience: de la perspective développementale, du pouvoir de la dynamique familiale, de la trajectoire contrariée vers l'indépendance individuelle et la formation de l'identité, des vicissitudes de l'expérience d'apprentissage. L'expérience d'avoir également travaillé avec des enfants plus jeunes fournit aux thérapeutes une appréciation différente des constellations défensives ainsi qu'une conscience nuancée des dynamiques de transfert lorsque les différences d'âge et de statut entre le praticien et le client sont plus marquées. Travailler avec des jeunes nécessite également une compréhension sophistiquée des dynamiques organisationnelles – qui sont moins enseignées dans les formations centrées autour de l'accompagnement des adultes. Ces éléments fournissent une perspective significativement différente sur le travail ce qui suggère donc que les apports d'une formation spécialisée sont d'une grande valeur. Des exemples sont fournis en guise d'illustration.

Εκπαίδευση στη συμβουλευτική νέων – τι προστίθεται από την ειδικότητα για παιδιά και εφήβους

ΠΕΡΊΛΗΨΗ

Η εργασία με μεγαλύτερους εφήβους και νεαρούς ενήλικες είναι μια διφορούμενη περιοχή. Αυτοί που έχουν δεξιότητες στην εργασία με ενήλικους, μπορούν εύκολα να προσαρμοστούν στην εργασία και με αυτήν την ηλικιακή ομάδα, και ιστορικά αυτή είναι η πιο συνηθισμένη διαδρομή για το ρόλο. Σε αυτό το άρθρο υποστηρίζω, ωστόσο, ότι υπάρχει πιθανότητα διαφοράς μεταξύ της προσέγγισής αυτών και εκείνων που έχουν εκπαιδευτεί εξειδικευμένα για να εργαστούν με παιδιά και εφήβους. Τέτοιες εκπαιδεύσεις είναι πιθανό να διανθίσουν στους επαγγελματίες μια μεγαλύτερη ευαισθητοποίηση για: την αναπτυξιακή προοπτική, τη σημασία των συνεχών οικογενειακών δυναμικών, την αμφιλεγόμενη πορεία προς την ατομική ανεξαρτησία και το σχηματισμό ταυτότητας, και τις ιδιαίτερες διακυμάνσεις της μαθησιακής εμπειρίας. Η εμπειρία της συνεργασίας και με μικρότερα παιδιά παρέχει στους συμβούλους/θεραπευτές μια διαφορετική εκτίμηση των αμυντικών καταιγισμών και μια διαφοροποιημένη επίγνωση της προβολής δυναμικών όταν η διαφορά στην ηλικία και θέση μεταξύ του επαγγελματία και του πελάτη είναι μεγαλύτερη. Η συνεργασία με νεότερους ανθρώπους απαιτεί επίσης μια εκλεπτυσμένη κατανόηση των δυναμικών σε οργανωτικό επίπεδο - οι οποίες είναι λιγότερο πιθανό να εμφανίζονται σε εκπαιδεύσεις ενηλίκων. Αυτά τα χαρακτηριστικά παρέχουν μια πολύ διαφορετική προοπτική στην εργασία, υποδηλώνοντας ότι η συμβολή εξειδικευμένης εκπαίδευσης έχει μεγάλη αξία. Στο άρθρο δίνονται παραδείγματα που επεξηγούν αυτές οι ιδέες.

PALABRAS CLAVE Jóvenes adultos; Formación; Adolescencia; Desarrollo Emocional; Aprendizaje y Enseñanza

PAROLE CHIAVE giovani adulti; formazione; adolescenza; sviluppo emotivo; apprendimento e insegnamento

MOTS-CLÉS jeunes adultes; formation; adolescence; développement émotionnel; apprendre et enseigner

ΛΈΞΕΙΣ ΚΛΕΙΔΙΆ Νέοι ενήλικες; Εκπαίδευση; Εφηβεία; Συναισθηματική Ανάπτυξη; Μάθηση και Διδασκαλία

(For ethical reasons, all examples used for illustration in this paper are based on amalgamations and/or fictionalised versions of real cases.)

In recent years there has been a marked increase in concern about the mental health of young adults, particularly on the perceived shortfall of provision in services for university and college students, with rising alarm about suicides and self-harm. As reported in the Guardian 27 September 2019b,

> 'British universities are experiencing a surge in student anxiety, mental breakdowns and depression. There has been a sharp rise in students dropping out – of the 2015 intake, 26,000 left in their first year, an increase for the third year running – and an alarming number of suicides. In the 12 months ending July 2017, the rate of suicide for university students in England and Wales was 4.7 deaths per 100,000 students, which equates to 95 suicides or about one death every four days.' Guardian (2019a)

In addition, '[i]n 2015/16, 15,395 UK-domiciled first-year students disclosed a mental health condition – almost five times the number in 2006/07. This equates to 2% of first-year students in 2015/16, up from 0.4 per cent in 2006/07' (Thorley, 2017, p. 1 of summary).

Demand for mental health support among young people is very high, with agencies serving this population struggling to keep up. '94% [of universities] report an increase in demand for counselling services, while 61% report an increase of over 25%. In some universities, up to 1 in 4 students are using, or waiting to use, counselling services' (Thorley, 2017). Some services have faced a 50% rise in referrals and there is widespread concern about waiting times (Guardian Newspaper, 2019b). Universities have put more public emphasis on both prevention, through wellbeing interventions at an early stage of distress, and on access to focussed mental health support, albeit with severe limitations on what can be made available. Some universities are increasing funding for wellbeing and counselling services; at Bristol, spending doubled from 2016 to 2017.

However, in all the discussions and concern around this much needed area of mental health support, there is rarely much, if any, emphasis on what kind of training is the most appropriate for those working with this age group. In this paper I discuss why a child and adolescent training can provide a different, and, I would argue, highly relevant set of skills and understandings which support high-quality work with this client group.

Historically, the majority of those working in higher and further education counselling services, and with the 18–25 year old age group more generally, have been trained on courses aimed primarily at adult work, rather than specialist courses or those concentrating on child and adolescent clients. (It remains the case that a large majority of counselling trainings are still focussed on work with adults, although the number of specialist child and adolescent trainings has increased in the last decade or so.) It is not difficult to argue that those counselling young children might need specialist training, as working using play, art and understanding of behaviour is so different from work where talking is almost the only means of communication (see Kegerreis, 2006). Even so, until recently this was not widely recognised in the counselling world and there were few opportunities to train in a dedicated course, especially if one was psychodynamically orientated. The longer and more intense psychotherapy trainings were mostly divided along age-group lines, but counselling with children was apparently considered something one became proficient at through experience, supervision and top-up CPD rather than with a core specialised training. More recently the BACP has developed excellent guidelines on competencies to demonstrate the specific skills required and to assist trainings in developing good programmes, (BACP, 2019) but there are still relatively few fully developed programmes available.

It is therefore not surprising that it is even more the case that late adolescents and young adults are provided with services in which most of the counsellors are trained in adult work. After all, words are the primary medium of communication, the young people are not usually seen in the context of and under the auspices of their family and in most cases, especially in HE, they are formally adults anyway being over 18. However, I will endeavour to show why and how a training in child and adolescent counselling offers key insights and skills which help in working with this age group. This is not to say that adult-trained counsellors cannot do an excellent job – of course they can – but it is to suggest that the difference in the trainings might lead to an approach to the work from a specific angle and call upon different resources, and that when working with a young adult there is great value in having worked with younger children and adolescents.

Adolescents, young adults or emerging adults?

Before continuing with this argument, it is worth pausing for a while to consider who these young people are. We can agree on a general age-range, but there are interesting issues of definition and description. Adolescence, if viewed from the perspective of therapeutic training, often includes patients as old as 21 or 25, even though people in this age-range are obviously at a very different life-stage than that of a 14 or 15 year old. But within popular culture there are significant sectors where the label of 'young adult' is applied even to the younger age-range (e.g., Young Adult fiction) with the lower end as young as 13. From Erikson (1950) onwards there have been important explorations of the particular tasks and features of those in this intermediate phase, and debate about a useful demarcation and appropriate label (See Keniston 1971; Levinson 1978). Building on these and other theorists, Arnett (2000) helpfully identifies this period as 'emerging adulthood' and details the distinctive features of this phase, which is neither adolescence nor adulthood. It is important to note, he says, that there is more diversity in this period than at any other, as it is 'a period when change and exploration are common' with 'heterogeneity one of emerging adulthood's distinguishing characteristics', 'a period in which many different potential futures remain possible and personal freedom and exploration are higher for most people than at any other time'(p. 479).

In terms of diversity of experience, there are clearly many differences between those in this age-range who are pursuing higher or further education and those who are not. This paper was written primarily for those working in further or higher education institutions, so it is these who are most in mind. However, despite the differences, many of the issues discussed are just as relevant to those pursuing other ways forward in their lives.

Training: The developmental perspective

Returning to the argument about what constitutes the most useful training with emerging adults, the first most crucial difference between an adult or child/adolescent orientated training relates to the depth of understanding of and breadth of experience gained in child and adolescent emotional development. Working with children of all ages gives us intimate knowledge of the age and stage-related challenges which face them along the way. We will have accompanied some children on their developmental journey from early childhood through latency, and will have worked with others through puberty and early adolescence. The emerging adult is only just moving on from – or is maybe still very much immersed in – these tumultuous changes, and their maturational journey remains very much a work in progress. If we have pursued an adult-orientated training we will know a considerable amount about this intellectually, but we would not have lived through it alongside clients each struggling with their own particular version of growing up.

If we have trained in child and adolescent work we are likely to have met younger adolescents who find the developmental tasks of puberty and adolescence overwhelmingly difficult. Some, like Sally-Anne, 15, develop serious psychosomatic symptoms (e.g., panic attacks with fainting and chest pains) while Connie (16) developed an eating disorder. In treatment, it became evident that with both clients their symptoms could be usefully understood to be desperate unconscious attempts to 'slam on the brakes' and refuse to become adult individuals, as this would mean leaving childhood behind and embarking on sexual lives. On the other hand, Marta (15) managed her conflicts by attempting to morph into an instant adult, finding the company of others of her age annoying and talking/acting in a very pseudo-mature way. She leapt into her sexual life as if without a care, while burying severe panic and insecurity in counter-phobic nonchalance and projecting anxiety into the adults who cared for her. The older young adults we work with may, or may not, be further on in their development as sexual beings, but having worked with and understood in depth the earliest stages of this in our clients can help so much in helping then navigate in these turbulent waters.

The perspective one gets working with children is different. With them we have the developmental drive in our favour, and our work can often be seen as trying to clear away obstacles that have arisen to normal processes rather than attempting major repair work on damaged pasts. We do not have the same rigidity of defences to deal with, there is less for our clients to regret, and identity is still fluid. The focus can be more on what is preventing normal development rather than on established and perhaps relied-upon dysfunctional structures. As I wrote in an earlier paper 'moving on to the next stage of life may be rendered impossible by the level on anxiety aroused or by the way in which it has not yet been possible to master the challenges of the earlier stage' (Kegerreis, 2006). Having these elements in mind helps a great deal when working with those a little later on in the process, while still not yet having settled into adult life.

The real and the phantasy family

Another key feature is a rich understanding of the real families involved – rather than the internalised family of an adult. If we are working with young adults in an educational setting, many of our clients will still be living in their family home or will return to it and their families in vacations, and crucially they are to a large extent likely to be still financially dependent on their parents. Unlike most adult clients, they do not have an establishment of their own which gives them at least notionally the possibility of choice over the distance or otherwise they can make with their families and the roles available to them. This means that the emotional difficulty of establishing oneself as an independent individual is compounded by the external reality of still being part of the original family at a practical level, which builds in greater power to the hold on us of those original projective dynamics. For example, Sasha, (21) a client in higher education, had worked hard in therapy to put some distance between her and her parents' highly conflictual relationship, into which she was continually drawn. When she first came to therapy while still in school she could not resist getting involved in their rows, taking her father's side very often and treating her mother to sometimes withering contempt, while also taking on a burdensome role to 'fix' what was going wrong with them one way or another, even if this meant convincing them to separate. In the year leading up to her going to university she was able to free herself considerably from this, and make a good start at leaving them to sort things out for themselves. However, coming back in the vacations faced her with a powerful tug back into this role, especially on one occasion when she found herself struggling with a romantic relationship which had not worked out as well as she had hoped. We had to work hard again on helping her extricate herself from her Oedipal dynamics.

Young adults are in the process of moving their centre of emotional gravity away from the family – into their friendship groups and into partnerships of their own. They need to find ways of belonging that are dependent on what they do and how they are, setting up networks of projective dynamics with others of their own choosing, which involves complex manoeuvres to work out how to manage many different parts of themselves. In our families of origin, we will have been heavily impinged upon and shaped by the projective needs of our parents and siblings. Once we are choosing for ourselves which people to spend time and emotional energy with we have to sort out our own emotional capacities and perhaps regain elements which have been precluded at home. If as a counsellor one has worked with younger children and with real ongoing family relationships, including often working with families rather than just individuals, one's toolkit and skill in using it is likely to be much more effective in helping with this.

We are also likely to be more closely attuned to the issues of where our young adult's development fits into the family life-cycle? What does separation and maturation mean for this specific young person and for their parents or siblings? For example, Gary, (18) was the first child from his family to leave home, which meant he was carrying both exaggerated hopes and fears from the family. In counselling, it was possible to gain insight into how he was weighed down by the burden of signifying for the parents the 'proof' of their success or failure as parents. For Nadia, her issue was that she was carrying the double-edged sword of going further in her career than her parents had done. Even though she was lovingly supported by their parents, there was an admixture of envy and even resentment at her successes.

Does doing well mean surpassing their families, which might lead to conflicts over loyalty and belonging? This, for some, can have powerful class, cultural and racial dimensions as well. Gaining further or higher education could signify moving away from their social group, renouncing certain identifications, and risking not fitting in any more or being perceived as having left their families behind. Carole, an afro-caribbean student on a counselling training, reported vividly how much of a struggle this was for her, as her pursuing the training was seen as a betrayal, an attempt to join white culture. She felt very isolated from her family and social group as a result. Envious attack might be a real possibility, but even without it a gulf can open up and it might be difficult to sustain progress if there is guilt about leaving parents/siblings behind and fear of getting 'lost'.

A further corollary of having worked with children and their real families, is that we are much more likely to have a deep awareness of the power of real family dynamics, having seen them in action. There is a caricature of the Kleinian approach in which the destructiveness can always be located in the client, with the focus squarely on their difficulties in making use of a good object, rather than the impact on them of damaging dynamics. At the other end of the spectrum, there are approaches in which the parents can readily get cast as the source of any if not all the difficulties and the client's own contribution is overlooked or perhaps too leniently considered. If in our training we have worked with *real* families, we will have seen real damage being done to our clients before our eyes, but on the other hand we will also have witnessed caring parents working very hard to do their best for a child who seems to resist their best endeavours. If we work with real families we are more likely to be able to get a balanced sense of the way in which relationships are co-created, and a nuanced awareness of how problems are caused, sustained and also ameliorated.

Working with primitive defences

Alongside taking fully on board the impact of the actual and ongoing family dynamics, on a child-focussed training there will also be an intense concentration on very early life and its vicissitudes, not only in theory but also by virtue of experiencing in direct work both how small children develop difficulties and how they employ defences to manage their emotional pain. That little child is only a little below the surface in fully mature clients, to be sure, but this is even more true in the case of young adults.

Working with young children who become destructive or self-destructive in their behaviour helps us think deeply about primitive defences, in which action is resorted to rather than thought or more neurotic manoeuvres. Kemal (9), for example, would throw cars at his counsellor and tip furniture over when he could not get her to give in to his wishes, and Talia would climb onto a cupboard when she wanted to assert how she was 'above' her counsellor when she needed to make her feel like the small one. On a more serious level Kiani (9) had been through a series of failed fostering placements and – in a desperate attempt on the one hand to find adequate containment and on the other to retain some sense of agency and control, seemed hell-bent on destroying the capacity of his counsellor or anyone to manage her destructive behaviour. If we have worked with this kind of acting out we might be much better placed to understand why Simone, herself adopted, as a college student on a humanities course acted so provocatively with tutors, missing many appointments, refusing to comply with expectations, more or less daring staff to ask her to leave, flaunting her disdain for them and for the educational process in which she had enrolled. Again, an adult-trained counsellor would most likely be able to help Simone, but her compulsive need to test boundaries and to both project and risk provoking her own rejection will be much more familiar to the child-trained counsellor who might have helped several 9 or 10 -year old 'Simone's.

Learning as an emotional relationship

The example of Simone brings forward how much working with younger children throughout their educational journey gives us insight into the complexity of the learner's relationship with their teachers, subject and academic abilities, i.e. an intimate knowledge of the emotional aspects of learning. All students will have complex transference dynamics involved in their relationship with their tutors, the university or college as a whole, their subject of study, experts in their field and their peers. If we are working with higher or further education students, even if well past the age of maturity, this understanding of the vicissitudes of being a learner, and of the many ways of defending against anxieties experienced in learning, will be of great value. While learning and inhibitions in relation to it can clearly be understood using the same kind of insight as an adult counsellor uses with difficulties adults face in their work and relationship with employment, there are also key differences.

The capacity to learn can be inhibited in so many ways (Kegerreis, 2010; Youell, 2006). We will all have met students like Sami, (23) who despite being bright and able, sabotaged his engagement with his studies by avoidance tactics such as procrastination and denial, failing to produce assignments, delaying his contact with his placement, not preparing for seminars or engaging productively with texts. Farzhad (19) could not make good use of seminars or experiential learning – in part as a result of a history of being shamed in his family for not knowing, but at the other end of the spectrum Felicity was paradoxically constrained in her contributions because deep down she was too afraid of her wish to humiliatingly outshine everyone else in the class – in other words she was too competitive and afraid of envy to speak. Students can be crippled by fear of failure or held back by fear of what success might mean and bring with it. Being able to learn involves a relationship with dependency, taking in from others, managing envy, coping constructively with rivalry, accepting the reality of one's 'junior' status and above all a faith in one's inner digestive and creative processes, all of which are often seriously jeopardised by difficulties in early life. Working with younger children as they process these difficulties and struggling to develop these capacities helps enormously in the understanding of how and why young adult students cope with academic demands.

As we all know, writing essays or producing other course work is a hugely challenging emotional task as well as an academic one. Mustering the hope, confidence and assertiveness needed to study and produce assignments can be a huge challenge. Taking in and relating successfully to what others have written on a subject, and then using one's own confidence and creativity to marshal an argument of one's own, involves complex Oedipal dynamics (see Barwick, 2000). Envy and/or rivalrous feelings can easily make it hard to read the work of others, and an ego-dystonic superego can attack our capacity to identify and value our own opinions and choose good examples of our own. Finding one's own voice as well as understanding and valuing the contributions that have gone before involves a benign relationship with one's inner objects and oneself, which is often elusive, as well as a good enough transference to the 'parents' as represented by the leading writers in our field (Spurling, 2008). If we have worked through these issues from the beginning of a child's relationship with learning and helped clear away these obstacles in their early stages we will have developed a much more intimate understanding of what might be getting in our young adult client's educational success.

The future

Furthermore, successful learning, just like successful therapy, involves an investment in one's own future – and child and adolescent work helps us tune into just how compromised and problematic our clients' relationships with this as yet totally unknown future is likely to be, particularly if they have had difficult early lives. With adults, we are obviously also working with the future, but this future has already taken some kind of shape, important choices and compromises have already been made and much more has become established, whether helpfully or unhelpfully. The emphasis may well be more about shedding the past or at least coming to terms with it, and working out how to let go of what is getting in our way, rather than dealing with the fears, hopes, fantasies and phantasies about the future (Mak-Pearce, 2005). Of course, with children and adolescents one is also working with the impact of the past, but there is more fluidity in the system. This can be helpful but on the other hand there is also much more likelihood that the future is frighteningly – and/or excitingly – open. These young people do not know *at all* whether they can make it in the real world. They have less to regret, which makes it easier to make changes (Kegerreis, 1985) but on the other hand they have no certainty whatsoever that they can manage adult life. The adolescent mindset is often one of extremes, so with young adults too there can be exaggerated hopes of idealised futures (fame, riches, acclaim) and at the same time exaggerated fears of visible disaster (shame, collapse, failure, loneliness, humiliation). For example, Colin (20) oscillated between grand fantasies of millionaire status with his start-up plans and crushing visions of poverty and homelessness, neither of which were very likely, but both of which protected him from a deeper fear – often a very powerful one for adolescents – of having to work hard without necessarily being all that noticeable or out of the ordinary. With nothing yet established to give ballast to these flights of imagination, the young person is emotionally connected to the future in a very different way from an adult, whatever course their life has taken thus far.

Responsibility and self-care

Furthermore, young adults are at the beginning of having to take full responsibility for themselves. This process has already started by the time we might be working with them but it is by no means completed, (if indeed it ever is -this can be a life-long struggle for us all). The thrill and allure of independence clash with the longing to be looked after, and the very real power suddenly handed to the young adult to make or break their own lives can be overwhelming. This capacity to do well or badly by ourselves is in itself the most powerful weapon of all to use in any troublesome dynamic with our parents, as well as being the arena for all our acting out and protest in relation to our own internal conflicts. Taking good 'parental' care of ourselves involves having internalised this from others, which might be highly compromised by earlier experiences of poor care, but it also involves a hugely generous act of forgiveness for real or perceived past wrongs. If we are carrying grievances from our childhood – as we all do to some extent – then doing well by ourselves may be beyond us, at least until we get to the point where we can forgo punishing our parents and give them the gift of taking pride in our achievements. For most this is conflictual, for some highly challenging.

If one has become experienced in working with adolescents grappling with these complex processes it is easier to connect with and work with how an 18–25 year old to manage what can still be a very early stage in this aspect of their development as adults. Patrice (20) was drinking heavily and getting into risky social/sexual encounters. She was defiant and contemptuous towards anyone she thought had judgmental views about this and declared forcefully that she was not going to regret any of it. She projected all anxiety about what she was doing into those around her, including of course her counsellor, but could not own it herself. It became clear in the work that for her to take a more responsible parental role in relation to herself, as well as creating anxiety she did not feel able to manage, would involve forgiving her parents, particularly her father, for what she felt had been neglect and a favouring of her younger sister. The counsellor was able to work well with this and help her move towards better self-care, aided by her deep understanding of how difficult these psychic manoeuvres can be as we move out of childhood.

The superego and ego-ideal

Another way of considering the young adult's negotiation either of ideas of the future or the capacity for self-care is to register that these inevitably involve the nature of and the relationship with the superego and the ego ideal. In adolescence this is often the area of most intense turmoil and volatility. As I wrote in 2014 ... '[y]oung people can become obsessively dominated by a horrific caricature of a conscience, buried in excruciating self-hatred, viciously critical self-consciousness and a particular kind of despair about themselves. It is during this period, as they take on board the need to take on their part in the wider world, that the destructive superego can become a ghastly, sometimes deadly, internal antagonist' (p. 14).

While we hope that having aspirations and a realistic ego-ideal will spur our young people on to make the most of their lives at this crucial stage, we also know only too well that their most pressing problems are often related to a deeply disturbed and unhelpful relationship with a punitive superego and an unattainable ego-ideal.

Creative use of these complex dynamics and imagined futures can be a key skill in work with young people, and will be one which can be more keenly developed if one has worked with it in the earlier stages.

'Reading' adolescents – problems of assessment

A great deal of what has been written above could be subsumed under a different title – 'reading adolescents accurately'. If we accept that young adults may still be heavily affected by the dynamics of the adolescent process, then it is not hard to see that an in-depth understanding of adolescence, more than that likely to be gained in an adult training, is likely to be of real importance.

Recent neurological research has taught us a great deal about the developing brain. As well as giving us vital insights into the earliest phases of brain development it has shed light on the major changes in the brain which take place in adolescence. We are very familiar with the emotional and hormonal upheavals of this stage of life, and of the states of mind which seem to powerful at this time, but now we also have a window into the neurobiological corollary of these in the brain (Music, 2011). The major reorganisation that is going on at brain level (Blakemore and Choudhary 2006) is becoming more fully understood and it has added a further layer of insight into what adolescence really means. This level of understanding has implications for how we can help our adolescent clients accept and adapt to what is happening, and can help us gauge more successfully the level of disturbance in our clients.

Making a sensible assessment of our adolescent or young adult client is sometimes very difficult. They can have a highly melodramatic way of expressing themselves, with mood-swings which would be deemed close to warranting clinical diagnosis of bipolar disorder in a later adult. They can also have a way of experiencing time which is different and sometimes problematic. For example, Jonno (18) would reassure his counsellor that he had stopped his drug-use, having not smoked 'for ages'. It took her a while to realise that these 'ages' turned out to be at most 2 weeks. In another example, Jamila seemed more like a small child in her appreciation of time, meaning that the month before her exam was to her such an enormous stretch of time that urgency about revision had no traction.

As we all know, adolescents can be impulsive, as the drive to express huge new energies is not yet tempered by the development of more self-control. (This natural observation is now supported scientifically by the scans which show that the regions connected with impulsivity and self-control develop last of all.) Action can often feel less frightening than self-reflection and is a ready-to-hand manic defence against sadness or depression. As they struggle with their identity, their sexuality and their new power to affect the lives of themselves and those around them, they can feel extremely potent at one moment and crushed by powerlessness and shame the next. This elasticity can mean that they can appear resilient while being highly at risk. We face twin dangers: of overreacting to their dramatic all-or nothing presentation, or of under-reacting, not fully tuning into how deeply vulnerable and dangerously self-destructive their state of mind can be. Accurate risk-assessment of adolescents is another skill which is likely to be more highly developed if we train with adolescents through this turbulent process.

Working with adolescents (Kegerreis, 2014; Phillips, 2011) is challenging and rewarding, but never easy. Skilful assessment of young adults will be much more likely to develop if one has acquired the confidence to navigate this territory on many occasions during one's training.

Transference and power dynamics

A further element in the work with which we are likely to be much more familiar and adept with is the nature of transference dynamics between the young adult and ourselves in the counselling. We need to tune in accurately to who the client feels they are with when they are with us, and this is likely to be closer to the experience of being a *child with an adult* than is the case with two adults. The transference is therefore even more immediately imbued with parental/authority links more than is the case with adults, even if these dynamics are bound to be present or to become established over time.

The age and stage difference between us will carry great power and will have multiple specific meanings to our younger client. In their eyes we have crossed many of the thresholds and passed many of the tests which still await them. With adult clients there will be many facets to how we are perceived by virtue of our chosen profession and their ideas of what it stands for. By some we may well be seen as more successful, having had a professional training and establishing ourselves in a way which is valued by society. By others we will be seen as having made very different choices from them, opting for a low-paid profession rather than pursuing more conventional wealth and success. Consciously and unconsciously they will be responding to their adult understanding of the path we have taken, and will be having emotional reactions to this in the light of how it compares with their own.

Some of these latter dynamics will be operating with our young adult client, but their own path has not yet taken shape, so there will be different projections into our standing in relation to their own and a different power dynamic in the room. As Mak-Pearce (2005) states, adolescents are very powerfully engaged in issues of status, with grand fantasies of changing the world one minute and a sense of being utterly insignificant the next. The way in which we are experienced as adults first, counsellors second, has an important effect on the dynamics of the counselling relationship which we might not be fully tuned into if we are used to working with older adults.

Furthermore, we are more closely identified with the institution, at least if the counselling is linked to their educational setting. There will be transferences to the organisation itself, which enter the counselling room, and again the more experience we have in metabolising and negotiating this the better we are likely to 'read' the situation.

Group and organisational dynamics

Children and adolescents are usually identified as belonging to groups and organisations, even more than is the case with adults. They spend their days in classrooms, impinged upon by and playing their own part in group dynamics, and these are themselves elements in complex institutions with their own organisational anxieties and defences. As children do not yet have families of their own their identification within these groups is likely to be of far greater importance to them than might be the case later in life.

A good child and adolescent training will, as a result, usually contain more emphasis on understanding group and organisational dynamics, quite often including some acquaintance with group work itself even if this is not emphasised as part of the training. This means that we are likely to be more acutely attuned to the group and organisational dynamics affecting our young adult client. If we only work with individual adults, we are likely to see their groups and organisations through the prism of their own anxieties and defences and may be less well equipped to understand the complex projective dynamics at work in an educational institution or learning group. Again, as described above in the section on the family, the adult has, at least in theory, some autonomy over their attendance at work or their being in a certain job or role, but children and adolescents by necessity have a different relationship with their educational institution. Our young adults have more autonomy than a school pupil to be sure, and have the capacity to leave, but their relationship with the organisation, and the dynamics surrounding them in the learning group, might well be closer to that of a school than that of an employing organisation.

There will be implications for the counsellor too if they are working within an educational institution. No matter what our clinical setting, our counselling work is affected by the framework within which we function, but if we work within an organisation with its own, non-counselling-related primary task, such as in an EAP, our work has to be understood and navigated differently from work done in, say, a community counselling or health service. To work successfully in a university or college counselling service, we have to have a very good grasp of how our work aligns with and is understood within the overall educational primary task. The understanding of this gained in a child and adolescent training will be of enormous value.

Conclusion

There is no doubt that a good adult training equips counsellors to work well with young adults. All the key elements required in the work, such as the capacity to work with primitive defences and an understanding of the developmental perspective and the demands of learning will have been included. This paper is decidedly not arguing that such a training falls short, but is suggesting that a good child and adolescent training will both add extra ingredients and significantly strengthen others. It will enable trainees to build up even greater breadth and depth of understanding and develop further in their skill and resourcefulness in therapeutic intervention and technique.

While there could be many questions raised in relation to any simple statement that child and adolescent training is *better* as a foundation, it may nonetheless be useful to reflect on how *differently* one might work with a given client if one comes to the work from these different trainings. One's orientation to the client and their pasts is likely to be different in all the ways outlined in this paper. Our understanding of the client, our responses to them and our particular balance of support and challenge might differ.

If we have trained primarily with adults, good supervision and later CPD can provide many of the resources we need, so there are other ways of helping develop the particular skill-sets required of this kind of work. What is vital is that as we try to meet the growing need for good-quality work with this age-group, we think not just in terms of the sufficient provision of counselling services but also in terms of what training and professional development enable us to work most effectively with them.

Disclosure statement

No potential conflict of interest was reported by the author(s).

References

Arnett, J. J. (2000). Emerging adulthood: A theory of development from the late teens through the twenties. *American Psychologist, 55*(5), 469–480. https://doi.org/10. 1037/0003-066X.55.5.469

BACP. (2019). *Core competences for work with children and young people.* https:// www.bacp.co.uk/media/5863/bacp-cyp-competence-framework.pdf

Barwick, N. (2000). Loss, creativity and leaving home: investigating adolescent essay anxiety. In Barwick (Ed). *Clinical Counselling in Schools,* pp 159–174.

Blakemore, S.-J., & Choudhury, S. (2006). Development of the adolescent brain: Implications for executive function and social cognition. *Journal of Child Psychology and Psychiatry, 47*(3–4), 296–312. https://doi.org/10.1111/j.1469-7610.2006.01611.x

Erikson, E. H. (1950). *Childhood and society*. Norton.

Guardian Newspaper. (2019a, September 16).

Guardian Newspaper. (2019b, September 27).

Kegerreis, S. (1985). Getting better makes it worse: Obstacles to improvement in children with emotional and behavioural difficulties. *Maladjustment and Therapeutic Education, 3*, 20–42. reprinted in Trowell, J. and Bower, M. (1996) *The Emotional Needs of Young Children and their Families, 1*(3), 102–108 London: Routledge.

Kegerreis, S. (2006). Working with children and adolescents – Is specialist training necessary? *Psychodynamic Practice, 12*(4), 403–418. https://doi.org/10.1080/14753630600958320

Kegerreis, S. (2010). *Learning: The hardest task of all in Psychodynamic counselling with children and young people*. Palgrave Macmillan.

Kegerreis, S. (2014). Working with Adolescents. Chapter 1. In French & Klein (Eds.), *Working with the child within, vol 2: The contemporary adolescent*, pp 7–18. Routledge.

Keniston, K. (1971). *Youth and dissent: The rise of a new opposition*. Harcourt Brace Jovanovich.

Levinson, D. J. (1978). *The seasons of a man's life*. Ballantine.

Mak-Pearce, G. (2005). *Community-based psychotherapy with young people* (G. Baruch, Ed.). Brunner- Routledge, Taylor & Francis Group.

Music, G. (2011). *Nurturing natures*. Psychology Press.

Phillips, A. (2011). The pleasures of working with adolescents. *Psychodynamic Practice, 17*(2), 187–197. https://doi.org/10.1080/14753634.2011.562698

Spurling, L. (2008). On psychoanalytic figures as transference objects. *The International Journal of Psychoanalysis, 84*(1), 31–43. https://doi.org/10.1516/YA50-U3H8-F19A-VQCN

Thorley, C. (2017). *Not by degrees: Improving student mental health in the UK's universities*. Institute for Public Policy Research. https://www.ippr.org/files/2017-09/not-by-degrees-summary-sept-2017-1-.pdf

Youell, B. (2006). *The learning relationship*. Routledge.

The narratives of parental alienation

Sally Parsloe

ABSTRACT

When families are in conflict, high levels of emotional activity such as anger, fear, loss and grief in the adults involved can affect children and young people in the family, particularly as a result of conscious and unconscious adult emotional pressure and manipulation. An aspect of this is when one parent uses their power over a child to excommunicate the other parent. This is sometimes called parental alienation. This terminology arises from the work of Richard Gardner, who developed the notion of Parental Alienation Syndrome. What lies behind the label parental alienation, the journey and implications of that phenomenon are explored. A consideration of the limitations of the UK court system reveals the lonely predicament of the child. This paper considers how psychotherapists may help young people to make sense of their experience of being caught up in destructive family narratives by claiming their own understanding and narrative.

Die Erzählungen der elterlichen Entfremdung

ABSTRACT

Wenn Familien in Konflikt geraten, kann ein hohes Maß an psychischer Aktivität wie Wut, Angst, Verlust und Trauer bei den betroffenen Erwachsenen Kinder und Jugendliche in der Familie betreffen, insbesondere aufgrund des bewussten und unbewussten emotionalen Drucks und der Manipulation von Erwachsenen. Ein Aspekt davon ist, wenn ein Elternteil seine Macht über ein Kind nutzt, um den anderen Elternteil zu exkommunizieren. Dies wird manchmal als elterliche Entfremdung bezeichnet. Diese Terminologie ergibt sich aus der Arbeit von Richard Gardner, der den Begriff des Parental Alienation Syndrome (Gardner, 1987, 1992) entwickelte. Was hinter dem Label elterliche Entfremdung steckt, die Reise und die Auswirkungen dieses Phänomens werden untersucht. Eine Betrachtung der Einschränkungen des britischen Gerichtssystems zeigt die einsame Lage des Kindes. In diesem Artikel wird untersucht, wie Psychotherapeuten jungen Menschen helfen können, ihre Erfahrungen mit destruktiven Familienerzählungen zu verstehen, indem sie ihr eigenes Verständnis und ihre eigene Erzählung beanspruchen.

Las narrativas de la alienación parental

RESUMEN
Cuando las familias están en conflicto, altos niveles de actividad psicológica como la ira, el miedo, la pérdida y el dolor en los adultos involucrados pueden afectar a los niños y jóvenes de la familia, particularmente como resultado de la presión emocional y la manipulación emocional de adultos conscientes e inconscientes. Un aspecto de esto es cuando uno de los padres usa su poder sobre un niño para excomulgar al otro padre. Esto a veces se llama alienación parental. Esta terminología surge del trabajo de Richard Gardner, quien desarrolló la noción de Síndrome de Alienación Parental (Gardner 1987,1992). Se explora lo que hay detrás de la etiqueta de alienación parental, el viaje y las implicaciones de ese fenómeno. Una consideración de las limitaciones del sistema judicial del Reino Unido revela la situación solitaria del niño. Este artículo considera cómo los psicoterapeutas pueden ayudar a los jóvenes a dar sentido a su experiencia de estar atrapados en historias familiares destructivas al pedir comprensión de su propia vivencia.

Le narrative dell'alienazione parentale

Quando le famiglie sono in conflitto sono elevati i livelli dell'attività psicologica, rabbia, paura, perdita e dolore negli adulti coinvolti possono influenzare i bambini e i giovani della famiglia, in particolare a causa della pressione e manipolazione emotiva e inconscia dell'adulto. Un aspetto di ciò è quando un genitore usa il proprio potere su un figlio per escludere l'altro genitore. Questo comportamento può essere chiamato alienazione genitoriale. Si tratta di un termine che deriva dal lavoro di Richard Gardner, che ha sviluppato la nozione di Sindrome da alienazione parentale (Gardner, 1987, 1992). Viene esplorato ciò che si nasconde dietro l'etichetta alienazione genitoriale, il percorso e le implicazioni di questo fenomeno. Una considerazione dei limiti del sistema giudiziario del Regno Unito rivela la situazione di solitudine del bambino. Questo articolo considera come gli psicoterapeuti possano aiutare i giovani a dare un senso alla loro esperienza di essere coinvolti in narrative familiari distruttive rivendicando il proprio pensiero e l'autonoma narrazione.

Histoires d'aliénation parentale

Lorsque les familles sont en conflit, des niveaux élevés d'activité psychologique telle que la colère, la peur, la perte ou le deuil des adultes peuvent affecter les enfants et les jeunes de cette famille, en particulier si c'est la résultante des pressions émotionnelles et de la manipulation des adultes, conscientes et inconscientes. Un des aspects est lorsqu'un des parents use de son pouvoir sur l'enfant pour excommunier l'autre parent. C'est ce qu'on appelle parfois l'aliénation parentale. Cette terminologie trouve son origine dans les travaux de Richard Gardner, qui a développé la notion de Syndrome d'Aliénation Parentale (Gardner, 1987,1992). Ce qui se cache sous cette étiquette d'aliénation parentale, le trajet et les implications de ce phénomène sont explorés dans cet article. Une considération des limites du système judiciaire britannique révèle la situation d'isolement des enfants. Cet article envisage ce que les psychothérapeutes peuvent mettre en place pour aider les jeunes à comprendre leur vécu d'être coincé dans une histoire familiale destructrice et favoriser leur propre compréhension et récit.

Τι διαφορά κάνεις. Μια φανταστική φαινομενολογία της συνεργασίας με έναν νεαρό ενήλικα

ΠΕΡΊΛΗΨΗ
Αυτό το άρθρο παρουσιάζει μια φανταστική φαινομενολογία της συνεργασίας με έναν νεαρό ενήλικα στην ψυχοθεραπεία. Η περίπτωση δείχνει τη σημασία της σιωπηρής και/ή ασυνείδητης «μετατόπισης» του νοήματος και της επικοινωνίας μεταξύ πελάτη και θεραπευτή. Ως θεραπευτές μπορεί να συναντήσουμε αυτό που ήταν απροσδόκητο σε εμάς στον πελάτη μας. Αυτό που αναδύεται είναι πτυχές του τρόπου με τον οποίο εξηγούμε/αντιλαμβανόμαστε αναδρομικά, οι οποίες διερευνώνται εν συντομία μέσα από τις αισθήσεις της διαφοροποίησης, της αποξένωσης, της καταστολής, της μυθοπλασίας και του θανάτου. Ο εξορθολογισμός και η επιστημονικοποίηση της εμπειρίας εισάγουν κάτι νεκρό. Διερευνάται η σημασία του να μιλάει ο πελάτης για τον εαυτό του. Οι νέοι ειδικά, φαίνεται ότι πρέπει να βρουν τη δική τους βιωματική γλώσσα, χωρίς να συνθλίβονται από τις λέξεις (και την παρουσία) των άλλων, αλλά το πώς αυτό είναι δυνατό μοιάζει δύσκολο.

PALABRAS CLAVE Jóvenes; niños; conflicto parental; alienación parental

PAROLE CHIAVE giovani; bambini; conflitto dei genitori; alienazione dei genitori

MOTS-CLÉS *Jeunes; enfantsconflit parental; aliénation parentale*

Λέξεις κλειδιά διαφοροποίηση; φαινομενολογία; μελέτη περίπτωσης; νεαρός ενήλικας; ψυχοθεραπεία; μυθοπλασία

Introduction

The author works therapeutically with people aged 17 and upwards and with family groups. She is also a lawyer and has represented children in court proceedings for many years. As a family mediator, she works with children involved in family breakdown. She has worked as a therapist with organisations that provide services for people estranged from family and who are caught up in family conflict.

This paper explores the way in which the narratives of adult conflict affect young people and it considers the various professional narratives that are used to seek to bring under control the discomfort of the adult world at the distress of children. One particular aspect of the acting out of adult conflict is taken as a lens through which to explore the means, dynamics and implications of ab-use of narrative. That aspect is a phenomenon that has been called parental alienation, discussed here as a weaponization of narrative that is claimed to have a particular shape, and a particular outcome, one which has attracted multidisciplinary concern, and which has been subject to targeted research which recommends more research. One might say it is a narrative about narrative that struggles to recognise the possibility of alternative narrative.

Parental alienation is an emotional action that has elicited controversy in the disciplines of the psychological therapies, family support services and legal professions across national boundaries. The term emotional action will be used in this paper to mean action in the emotional realm which arises from the conscious or unconscious, which may be manifested physically or verbally, or which may be non-verbal and 'sensed', but which has an impact on another person. Often, there is a desire to define and wrap phenomena in a labelled parcel, so that we can *know* just what's inside and what remedies may be applied. Unfortunately, parental alienation is an intransigent and complex problem, slippery to solution, and so it might be worth looking at it from a standpoint of perplexity, of not-knowing, thus seeing what emerges.

The author will start with a brief discussion of the history of legal and psychological thinking about this phenomenon and will then move to try to look underneath and beyond the narratives surrounding it. A case study helps to illuminate what it might be like for a young person caught up in the flak, revealing this playing out of adult conflict to be an emotional action that causes all sorts of problems for young people that can be really quite serious, the effects of which can often be seen in the therapeutic room but which are very strongly denied by the young person. This work, the author suggests, demands careful attention, as the defences of the client protect that which is extremely painful to the touch, and are thus commensurately active.

A brief story of parental alienation

The idea of an emotional action called parental alienation was first described by Wallerstein and Kelly in 1976. The label Parental Alienation Syndrome however was introduced by Richard Gardner, an American psychotherapist, on the basis of his observation of what happens and what results from parental conflict situations when one parent turns the child against the other parent by a misuse of their power over the child (Gardner, 1987, 1992). Gardner suggested that there was a constellation of phenomena that might be observed when working with young people that would indicate what he termed Parental Alienation Syndrome. These manifestations included a lack of sense of guilt in the child at the ostracism and denigration of the alienated parent, borrowed scenarios, absurd reasons for the denigration, a dissolving of the child's independent opinion, reflexive support of the alienating parent and lack of ambivalence.

Parental Alienation Syndrome is one of the few emotional conditions that has not been included as a label in the DSM. However, in a world in which it seems no human phenomenon can be left uncolonized by science, Parental Alienation *outcomes* are classified in the fifth edition of the *Diagnostic and*

Statistical Manual of Mental Disorders as a mental condition under the diagnosis 'child affected by parental relationship distress' (CAPRD; Bernet et al., 2016).

Gardner's classification of parental alienation as a syndrome was disputed by the legal and psychological community, arguably as a reaction to his controversial views on peadophilia (i.e, suggesting that while paedophilic behaviour was a bad thing, it was a part of the repertoire of sexuality, a human potentiality in us all, then as now an unpopular way of thinking about atypical sexual behaviour). In the UK legal system judges and other professionals often prefer to use the term Implacable Hostility, but this term does not cover precisely the same phenomenon (damaging though it is in itself). Whatever the label, and whatever Gardner's unpopularity, it was not possible to ignore that something particular was happening in terms of emotional action in some families, and considerable further research followed. That research seemingly superseded Gardner's work, but on analysis seems to re-reveal much of what Gardner found, retaining part of the label, drawing similar conclusions whilst putting Gardner's work and name into shadow. It is striking that the person whose work dealt with the erasure of the unpopular and threatening (one way of looking at parental alienation) was himself subject to an attempt at erasure from the story, an aspect discussed by Michael Bone (Bone, 2003).

A review and distillation of research contained in the 2018 Review Of Research And Case Law On Parental Alienation (Doughty et al., 2018) commissioned by a UK organisation called CAFCASS*1, led to the formulation of a 'set of tools' to help those involved in disputes involving children to gain a better understanding of how children experience the separation of their parents. Under the heading parental alienation, there is a particular tool recommended for analysing certain behaviours to see if they indicate parental alienation.

These behaviours, set out in the CAFCASS Child Impact Assessment Framework, are strikingly like those that Gardner identified and include:

Having an opinion of one parent that is unjustifiably one sided.

Vilifying the rejected parent.

Reactions that are disproportionate to behaviour

Speaking without prompting about the rejected parent's shortcomings

Revision of history or recollection of events that couldn't have been remembered.

No ambivalence to the rejected parent.

The child claims to be fearful, but is aggressive or belligerent about the rejected parent.

The effects of parental alienation as disclosed by research

The research of psychological therapists has found that where one parent turns the child against the other, it leads to negative long-term effects on the mental health of the child, such as lack of trust in others and lack of trust in the child's own feelings, low self-regard and depression, attachment and adjustment issues in relationships and generally a higher incidence of mental health issues (Baker, 2005; Baker & Ben-Ami, 2011). Baker (2005) found that the hatred of the alienated parent may be internalized as a hatred of self, as the child grows in the realisation that they have something of the alienated parent in them. In addition, the Baker and Ben-Ami study (Baker & Ben-Ami, 2011) found that the child participants internalized the alienating parent's message that the alienated parent did not love them and this made them feel unlovable.

Karen Woodall is a UK psychotherapist who works extensively with families in which parental alienation occurs. Woodall however chooses not to use the term parental alienation, she instead uses the term induced psychological splitting. She makes the observation that there is a split in young people's language which may be heard as manifestation of parental alienation so that for them, attuned to the non-verbal action of the alienating adult which demands that they act out what is unspoken, language becomes behavioural rather than symbolic (Woodall, 2020a). She found that this induced psychological splitting causes what Winnicott called the false self (Winnicott, 1960), the child alienated from itself, therefore having no knowledge that it does not have its own mind, convinced that its views about the alienated parent are its own (Woodall, 2020b).

The disabling of ambivalence

Research, including that of Gardner, and the conclusions of the CAFCASS Review, highlight lack of ambivalence as a factor arising in parental alienation situations.

'Specifically, the expressed lack of ambivalence as manifested by the alienated child serves as an observable defining characteristic of the presence of parental alienation'. (Jaffe et al., 2017).

Jaffe et al. (2017) and Corradi (2013) suggest that a way to view the implication of ambivalence (and lack of it) in the context of parental alienation may be in terms of Freud's Oedipal model. The ambivalence in the Oedipal situation gives rise to fear of violence in the shape of castration or patricide, which brooding potentiality is peacefully defused by identification with the same sex parent. This is a resolution in which no one has to die and a way in which relationships may be maintained with all the family players, despite it entailing a relinquishing of certain passions towards the opposite sex parent, which relinquishing carries regret, but is consensual. However, in parental alienation situations, the anxiety of ambivalence is only resolved by the child choosing one parent and rejecting the other, depriving the child of the opportunity to be simultaneously angry with and love a parent. Corradi (2013) suggests that the inability to tolerate simultaneously love and hate leads to 'a legacy of failure and abandonment expectations', a failure of trust, which acted out through transference is expressed in splitting. He observed that borderline and parentally alienated children share similar characteristics of object relatedness to specific love objects, and that splitting pushes borderline individuals to destroy relationships. One might say the same is true for the alienated child who is forced to deny the positive attributes of the alienated parent. Anna Freud (1966) pointed out that denial as a mechanism adversely affects the ability to learn from experience and thus to develop flexible coping mechanisms.

Going further, to the heart of things, the French psychotherapist and philosopher Jacques Lacan suggests that ambivalence is the cornerstone of psychoanalysis, that to have an unconscious inherently posits ambivalence. Instead of 'ambivalence' Lacan used the word 'hainamoration' (hateloveing), stating that one cannot have love without hate (Lacan, 1999, p. 91). Hainamoration constitutes an existential experience of a subject fundamentally split by language. We might then see something of the full disaster to the person when this fundamental experience is suppressed, or distressed.

Responses to parental alienation

The UK legal system (which must have regard to the 1989 Children Act, and currently to the United Nations Convention on the Rights of the Child) wrestles to harmonise the rights of children to participate in decisions made about them with the responsibility of the courts to make decisions that are 'in the best interest of the child'. It is judicially presumed that the best interest of the child is to have contact with both of their parents. Thus, a UK judge has a duty to promote contact between children and their parents. The CAFCASS review cites the words of the judge in Mabon v Mabon ([2005] EWCA Civ 634), that in safeguarding children's UNCRC rights, one has to accept (in the case of articulate teenagers) that the right to freedom of expression and participation outweighs the paternalistic judgment of welfare, but goes on to say that parental alienation poses a dilemma where adopting a children's rights perspective may be unhelpful if the child has been subject to the indoctrination of an alienating parent, yet in breach of their rights if they are forced into reunification with the alienating parent (Bala et al., 2010).

The CAFCASS review tabulates the kind of interventions which were the subject of research. These were:

(a) questionnaires given to families to identify parental alienation,
(b) 4 day workshops for families,
(c) a retreat for children away from both parents with psycho-educational input prior to the alienated parent joining the child where they both then receive psycho-educational input, with the alienating parent receiving therapy off-site,
(d) family group work with a focus on cognitive behavioural modules, coping strategies, 'new' life story work and expressing feelings,
(e) a five day family 'camp' run by pro-bono psychologists.

The CAFCASS Review states that lack of quantitative data makes meta-analysis of the research unviable. None of the studies, it says, would stand up to robust scrutiny from NICE*2. One might think that this leaves the legal professionals doing what they believe to be the best for children with little guidance in a complex area, not knowing what to do or what they are dealing with when faced with the implications for children of this particular emotional action of adults in conflict.

A 2019 case heard by the Family Court in the UK, Re H, was an example of a judge, assisted by the report of one of the leading experts on parental alienation, Dr Janine Braier, making a very thoughtful analysis of the factors that indicate parental alienation, the causes, and the effects. However, for every such case, there are probably hundreds that do not get the timely and considered analysis that occurred in Re H. Another case, Re A, tragically showed the irreparable effect of not identifying parental alienation at a sufficiently early stage, so that all the court could do was to conduct effectively a post-mortem over the body of the child's relationship with its alienated parent.

Despite the CAFCASS Review of research, Sir James Munby, former President of the Family Courts in the UK, in a speech given in February 2020 (Munby, 2020) called for a 'comprehensive international literature review of all the existing non-legal research into the existence, causes, and consequences, and means of identifying parental alienation'.

Barnett (2020, p. 18) comments that: "It's all very well to look at the reported cases in the study, but we really don't know what is going on in the thousands of cases in the lower courts. We need to know to what extent parental alienation is being alleged, whether it is justified, how it's being constructed and what its consequences are'.

While the psychological professionals dispute parental alienation, what it comprises and how to deal with it, a legal voice expressed a helpful suggestion. Mr Justice McFarlane, now President of the Family Division (that part of the UK judicial system that deals with Family cases), expressed the view that the courts must focus on the particular behaviour of the particular parent in relation to the particular child in each individual case. If the Family Courts can approach the plight of the child phenomenologically, one would hope that we as therapists can do so too.

A phenomenological account

Danny is 19. He went into therapy because he had had a disappointment and he needed some help. He had wanted since he was 14 to go into the Army and he had been rejected twice because he couldn't pass the written tests. He was suffering from panic attacks. When he went into exams, or tried to write an essay, all that he had learned went blank and he did not know what to say. He was unable to put a single word onto paper and this caused him to panic. Danny felt that in the panic attacks it was as if his mind was disappearing.

About his parents, he said 'My dad has provided all my parenting. My mum betrayed the family and I don't see her'. He recounted a story in which his mother and father had separated when he was 12 as a result of his mother having an affair. Despite his father's frequent attempts through the court system to obtain custody of him, Danny lived until he was 14 with his mother. However, then he recounted, his mother's new partner assaulted him and he had gone to live with his father. Danny used extremely harsh expressions for his mother (e.g. abusive, non-mother, adultress) and his animosity extended to her partner and her father, Danny's grandfather. In contrast, he called his father a hero. He had been a soldier and had served in Northern Ireland during the Troubles and Danny said that he had suffered mentally from it but that suffering was made worse by his mother's adulterous behaviour. Danny recalled his father's devastation when he discovered the adultery. He remembered his father crying and crying. This was awful for Danny to witness. Danny himself wept as he remembered. Danny volunteered that his father had not tried to influence his feeling, on the contrary, his father had allowed him to help prepare all the written statements his dad had made for the court. Danny himself had also made written statements against his mother and her new partner to various professionals including the police. He emphasised that this was not because his dad got him to, but because he had personally felt so strongly that he wanted to make the statements. His dad had helped him with the wording and sending them to the various professionals, but it was he, Danny, who had wanted to do it.

He said his mother was a liar. She kept on lying to him in the few contact visits there had been, saying that there had been no assault by her boyfriend.

She kept reminding him that the court had found that there had been no assault, but Danny railed against the court system and how it couldn't be trusted in the face of liars anyway. When asked, Danny himself said had no memory of the assault, he couldn't remember it, but he knew it had happened otherwise he would never have said it did, would he? Why would he? When he was asked to consider whether there might be two or even more viable versions of events, he became extremely agitated and angry with his therapist, and threatened to stop coming to sessions. The idea of differing perspectives had to be introduced very softly, noticing, in moments when he felt most contained and held in the therapeutic room, where he might have said something before which was a little bit different to what he was now saying, in terms of feeling or sense-making, so that difference could be experienced as non-threatening.

But the main thing, for Danny, was how he could get into the Army. He wanted to know what to say on the psychological tests. He was convinced there must be the right thing to say and became agitated because no one would tell him what to say. He said it wasn't what he wanted to say that mattered, it was what they wanted to hear and if he knew that he could say it.

He believed strongly that the British Army was a force for good. He was incensed about prosecution of British soldiers who had served in Ireland. He thought the stories had been concocted and were malicious falsehoods. He thought the people who made the allegations were motivated by their own agendas, people up the chain. He wished there was still the death penalty for people who made false allegations, because 'getting rid of the liars gets rid of the lies'.

One of the things Danny accused his mum of was not understanding him, and not having the capacity for loyalty or self-sacrifice. 'She doesn't want me to get into the Army, she thinks I might be killed, but she doesn't understand, that would be fine by me. It's part of the job, to lay down your life for your country'.

Approaching parental alienation through ideas of narrative

The work of Continental philosophers Lyotard (whose ideas about narrative became known as postmodern) and Levinas may offer a way of understanding Danny (for it is understanding that he is asking for, not the imposition of solution) and for thinking in a wider way about the situations of the many other young people caught up in this harmful adult manipulation of narrative, and how we too as practitioners get caught up in the grand narratives of power, fear and ostracism.

Lyotard writes in The Post Modern Condition,

I will use the term modern to designate any science that legitimates itself with reference to a metadiscourse … making an explicit appeal to some grand narrative, … I define postmodern as incredulity toward metanarratives.

(Lyotard, 1984, p. xxiv).

One might say that Danny had become so alienated that he didn't even know he was alienated. His beliefs were either strong, violent and intractable, or entirely absent, so that he couldn't find out from himself what he himself wanted to say, but looked instead to see what he should say. He was in some ways like a cracked mirror, certain reflections grossly exaggerated, others obscured completely. The idea of creating his own narrative, one which could accommodate inconsistency and variation according to mood, moment and experience was blocked from him.

Perhaps a helpful offering in our work with young people, particularly those involved in conflicts between adults whom they love and to whom they are attached, might be about allowing the young person to look at reflections from different mirrors, to experiment with their own voice, to allow ambivalence, inconsistency and incredulity. In this way, different meanings and the meaning of difference open up, and they can get an experience of sorting through a plurality of voices and truths. As Lyotard writes in Just Gaming (Lyotard & Thébaud, 1979, p. 47), 'We have to judge case by case", pointing to Aristotelian phronēsis or practical wisdom as a model, but without the overarching community telos as elucidated in Aristotle's (384–422 BCE) Nichomachean Ethics. One kind of practical wisdom in Danny's case might be working with him to restore the possibilities in ambivalence to help him make sense of the conflict in his life.

John C. Hoffman describes how Gardner, the early exponent of parental alienation, used story in therapeutic work with children who were suffering, on his description, Parental Alienation Syndrome (Hoffman, 1986). Exploration of narrative, in the radical possibility of speaking and being heard in the therapeutic room, also offers a medium for the young person to discern something of the implications of alterity. The mode of saying in Levinas' Otherwise than Being brings us, in all its performative energy, towards the immensity of the meaning of the face of the other, and reveals the call of responsibility. In order for this to happen, the saying needs to be witnessed as a gesture to another:

I still interrupt the ultimate discourse in which all the discourses are stated, in saying it to one that listens … That is true of the discussion I am elaborating at this very moment. (Levinas, 1974, p. 170)

The dilemma of adults and of children

As we have seen, too often a child is left with an alienating parent not as a result of careful consideration of each individual case, but simply because the issue is too complicated and demanding for a clogged court system to deal with, and too expensive in terms of legal fees for most parents to obtain. Therapeutic work with an alienated child still in the care of the alienating parent poses a serious challenge, or therapy may take place later, in adulthood, after the harm has solidified.

For many legal and psychological practitioners, as the research demonstrates, the aim of work with young people is to get them 'back' with the alienated parent. Given the harm done by alienation, one might fully understand why this approach is taken. However, one might suggest that it is worth considering that in a no-win situation, the child is not always a passive victim, but may be a responsible participant.

This would be a recalibration of the suggestion of Jaffe et al. (2017), citing a study on Stockholm Syndrome (De Fabrique et al., 2007), that it is the most powerful parent that wins the battle for hearts and minds. It might recognise that the child senses the fear and fragility of the alienating parent and so chooses some sort of lesser evil, or necessary sacrifice (present in Danny's holding of the sacrificial position). It might be too much for adults to acknowledge the child's lonely predicament of sacrificial choice, and the adult's denial of that opportunity to choose could be a violence to the child.

It is a totem that it is adults who take the decisions, but is this not an investiture that saves the parent, not the child (where parenthood is claimed as a prop in a version of authority)? Here, authority establishes authority and then abrogates it and allocates its helplessness to not enough authority, not enough intervention, and so on in its search for endless power masquerading as responsibility.

What cannot perhaps be faced is the impossibility of coming to a clear answer, a scalpel solution, that can cut discomfort out for both child and adult. In the phenomenon that is called parental alienation, where the adults don't know what to do, the question of the narrative of power comes round and round. The idea of leaving a child stuck with a murderous narrative about one parent is disturbing, and if the situation is tested in court an increasingly preferred outcome is a transfer of residence to the targeted parent. When the phenomenon is seen in the therapeutic room the focus of the work is often re-unification with the alienated parent. Analogies are drawn with scenarios of violent abduction, like Stockholm Syndrome, or where children are kept in lonely cellars with kidnappers who become their only source of identity and relationship. As we have seen, great harm ensues when a child is asked to hate and reject a parent, but one might form the view that great harm may also be caused by a forcible removal from a parent to whom a child is strongly attached partly as a result of that parent's inner fragility. Perhaps this is an area around which further research could be helpful.

So often, when working with young people caught up in adult conflict, the arena of the conflict is transferred into the child, just as it is in cases of what is called parental alienation. Therapeutic practice seems to show that there always results for the child the necessity of trying somehow to block out the shocking war-noise of the competing narratives by choosing one and eliminating all others but, if they can find a space that is reliable and open, they may slowly be allowed to make their own sense of different narrative strands, an idea that Gardner recognised early in the story. This, the author would suggest, can best be attempted by providing the safety to develop trust in their own narratives of experience, and thus their bases of existence. If these bases are eroded, the child has no compass point of reference and is destined to be forever tossed on the storms of others' emotional states. In speaking to young people in this situation, they can often evince an extreme sort of certainty, which is not theirs, and which can act as a concrete wall to ambivalence and individual truth, a wall that holds them inside, with highly fortified defences inside which grief and shame, remorse, fear and judgement reign. In making court orders that remove the child from the alienating parent, the intention is to provide respite from alienating narrative, in the hope that the targeted parent can provide a safe space for the child. Perhaps the therapy room could be used as a free space, if as therapists we can liberate ourselves from the narratives of power in which we are entangled. It is a trope of the Family Court process that the voice of the child must be heard. The same goes for the therapeutic room.

The author worked with a family in which the mother constantly in the adult sessions used abusive names about the father, and blamed him violently for all the family difficulties. Her vitriol and rage were palpable (he had actually let her down in many ways) and she couldn't control it. The mother said however that she told their 11 year old daughter that Dad loved her. She thought this let her off the hook from examining her own violent hatred of and behaviour towards the father, who sat in silent hopelessness through these onslaughts. The child was able to articulate in her own sessions the extent of the strain of her life, and desire for her parents to get on, but also said with much sadness, that she knew her mother would never forgive her father, and that she had to try to live between both of them. However, over the course of four months' work in therapy, it became harder and harder for her not to be drawn into the mother's narrative. In sessions, she talked about what was going on and what new horror the father had perpetrated upon the mother (according to mother) that week, but was able to examine it and create some sort of parallel narrative, to her evident relief. The child's condition of coming to sessions was that none of what she said should ever be relayed to her parents. After four months, her mother withdrew consent to the therapy continuing.

Recognitions rather than answers

What then do the thoughts of philosophers, the research of psychological practitioners, and the experience of working in the room disclose, through the lens of parental alienation, about weaponised narratives of power?

Can we recognise the violence to the young person of the adult world? Can we bear the notion that harm to children comes not only from murderous parents and paedophiles, but from the fantasy of the adult world that we can control it and make it better if only we have robust research, funding and power? This may lead to paying lip service to the importance of individual experience but then consigning it to the heap of other experiences so that it becomes indistinguishable. It is one thing noticing that a phenomenon occurs. It is another to give it a label and enter it in the DSM as a pathology, or in the case of the law, confined by the limits and excesses of its own power, to make draconian orders directly against the child's express wish.

On the other hand, what about recognition from the postmodern viewpoint that even from within that controlling paradigm, there might arise insights of value that can help in the room, like the fact that in the face of the impossibility of creating a world where young people are truly protected, things are being tried by people who are genuinely trying to help but who are themselves tied up in conflicting authoritarian ideas, perhaps going with the one that seems to carry most power at any given time so that at least something can be felt to be 'done'.

One young woman told me, in tears, ' I used to say to myself, you're my parents, why can't you just sort it out. Why do I have to do it?' Can we as adults bear to say, 'I am sorry, I am not sure I can make it better, but I hear how painful it is and I will listen. Would you like to say more?'

*1CAFCASS: The Children and Family Court Advisory and Support Service, which is the department of mainly social workers that assists the family courts in the UK.

*2 NICE: The National Institute for Health and Care Excellence (NICE) is a public body of the Department of Health in England which publishes guidelines in respect of health and social care. It uses primarily evidence-based evaluation in appraisals that form the basis of the formulations of the guidelines.

Disclosure statement

No potential conflict of interest was reported by the author(s).

References

Baker, A. L. (2005). The long-term effects of parental alienation on adult children: A qualitative research study. *The American Journal of Family Therapy, 33*(4), 289–302. https://doi.org/10.1080/01926180590962129

Baker, A. L., & Ben-Ami, N. (2011). To turn a child against a parent is to turn a child against himself: The direct and indirect effects of exposure to parental alienation strategies on self-esteem and well-being. *Journal of Divorce & Remarriage, 52*(7), 472–489. https://doi.org/10.1080/10502556.2011.609424

Baker, A. L., Burkhard, B., & Albertson-Kelly, J. (2012). Differentiating alienated from not alienated children: A pilot study. *Journal of Divorce & Remarriage, 53*(3), 178–193. https://doi.org/10.1080/10502556.2012.663266

Bala, N., Hunt, S., & McCarney, C. (2010). Parental Alienation: Canadian Court Cases 1989-2008. *Family Court Review, 48*(1), 164–179. https://doi.org/10.1111/j.1744-1617.2009.01296.x

Barnett, A. (2020). A genealogy of hostility: Parental alienation in England and Wales. *Journal of Social Welfare and Family Law, 1*(1), 18–29. https://doi.org/10.1080/09649069.2019.1701921

Bernet, W., Wamboldt, M. Z., & Narrow, W. E. (2016). Child affected by parental relationship distress. *Journal of the American Academy of Child and Adolescent Psychiatry, 55*(7), 571–579. https://doi.org/10.1016/j.jaac.2016.04.018

Bone, J. M. (2003, Fall/Winter). Parental alienation syndrome: Examining the validity amid controversy. *Commentator: The Family Law Section, XX*(1), 24–27. http://dx.doi.org/10.1080/01926180903586583

CAFCASS Child Impact Assessment Framework. CAFCASS. https://www.cafcass.gov.uk/grown-ups/professionals/ciaf/

Corradi, R. B. (2013). Ambivalence: Its development, mastery, and role in psychopathology. *Bulletin of the Menninger Clinic, 77*(1), 41–69. https://doi.org/10.1521/bumc.2013.77.1.41

De Fabrique, N., Romano, S. J., Vecchi, G. M., & Van Hesselt, V. B. (2007). Understanding Stockholm Syndrome. *FBI Law Enforcement Bulletin, 76*(July), 10–15.

Doughty, J., Maxwell, N., & Slater, T. (2018). Review of research and case law on parental alienation. *Commissioned by CAFCASS Cymru April 2018.*

Freud, A. (1966). *The ego and the mechanisms of defence.* The Hogarth Press.

Gardner, R. A. (1987). *The parental alienation syndrome and the differentiation between false and genuine sex abuse.* Creative Therapeutics, Inc.

Gardner, R. A. (1992). *The parental alienation syndrome: A guide for mental health professionals.* Creative Therapeutics, Inc.

Hoffman, J. C. (1986). *Law, freedom and story: The role of narrative in society, therapy and faith.* Wilfred Laurier University Press.

Jaffe, A. M., & Thakkar, M. J., & Pascale Piron | Peter Walla (Reviewing Editor). (2017). Denial of ambivalence as a hallmark of parental alienation. *Cogent Psychology,* 4(1). doi:10.1080/23311908.2017.1327144.

Kruk, E. (2011). *Divorced fathers: Children's needs and parental responsibilities.* Fernwood Publishing.

Lacan, J. (1999). *On feminine sexuality, the limits of love and knowledge. 1972–1973. Encore: The seminar of Jacques Lacan book XX.* (Ed. J-A Miller, trans. B. Fink). Norton.

Levinas, E. (1974). *Autrement qu'être ou au-delà de l'essence, The Hague: Martinus Nijhoff,* (Otherwise than Being or Beyond Essence, Alphonso Lingis (trans.)). Kluwer Academic Publishers.

Lyotard, J., & Thébaud, J.-L. (1979). *Au juste.* Christian Bourgois. 1979 (*Just Gaming,* translated Wlad Godzick, Minneapolis, MN: University of Minnesota Press, 1985).

Lyotard, J. F. (1984). *The post-modern condition: A report on knowledge.* University of Minnesota Press. Lyotard, J. F. (1989).

Munby, J. (2020). http://www.transparencyproject.org.uk/the-crisis-in-private-law-by-sir-james-munby/

Re H (Parental Alienation). (2019). EWHC 2723 (Fam) in Family Law Dec 2019 Lexis Nexis.

Wallerstein, J. S., & Kelly, J. B. (1976). The effects of parental divorce: Experiences of the child in later latency. *American Journal of Orthopsychiatry,* 46(2), 256–269. https://doi.org/10.1111/j.1939-0025.1976.tb00926.x

Winnicott, D. W. (1960). *"Ego distortion in terms of true and false self", in The maturational process and the facilitating environment,* (2018) Abingdon: Routledge. https://doi.org/10.4324/9780429482410.

Woodall, K. (2020a). https://karenwoodall.blog/2020/06/06/giving-voice-to-the-uspeakable-the-language-of-the-alienated-child/

Woodall, K. (2020b). https://karenwoodall.blog/2020/05/25/alienation-of-the-self-from-the-self-the-problem-for-children-induced-to-use-defensive-splitting/

What differend do you make? An imaginary phenomenology of working with a young adult

Tony McSherry

ABSTRACT

This article presents an imaginary phenomenology of working with a young adult in psychotherapy. It is presented in two parts: Part 1 is a retrospective of meaning, and Part 2 is the case itself. The case indicates the intertwining and uncertainty of experience in therapy through the subjectivity of the therapist, a phenomenon which gives rise to something therapeutic. In Part 1, what emerges after reading the case over are some aspects of how we attach meaning *in retrospect*, which are explored through senses of differend, alienation, repression, fiction, and death. The young client especially it appears needs to find his own language of experience, without being crushed by the words (and presence) of others, but how this is possible seems fraught with difficulty How do we provide a safe space for a young person to speak and find their own way without imposing the co-ordinates of our own lives upon them? Perhaps one way is to be prepared to let go of our firm beliefs and ideas, without rancour, in the face of the energy and curiosity of youth.

Welchen Unterschied machst du? Eine imaginäre Phänomenologie der Arbeit mit einem jungen Erwachsenen

ABSTRAKT

Dieser Artikel präsentiert eine imaginäre Phänomenologie der Arbeit mit einem jungen Erwachsenen in der Psychotherapie. Der Fall zeigt die Bedeutung stillschweigender und/oder unbewusster „Abweichungen" von Bedeutung und Kommunikation zwischen Klient und Therapeut. Als Therapeuten können wir durch den Klienten herausfinden, was in uns selbst unerwartet war. Was dabei herauskommt, sind Aspekte, wie wir im Nachhinein erklären/verstehen, die kurz durch die Sinne von Unterschied, Entfremdung, Unterdrückung, Fiktion und Tod untersucht werden. Rationalisierungen und Erfahrungsforschung führen etwas Totes ein. Die Wichtigkeit, dass der Klient für sich selbst spricht, wird untersucht. Besonders die jungen Menschen scheinen das Bedürfnis zu haben, ihre eigene Sprache der Erfahrung zu finden, ohne von den Worten (und der Anwesenheit) anderer niedergeschlagen zu werden, aber wie dies möglich ist, scheint mit Schwierigkeiten behaftet zu sein.

Las diferencias que se observan; Una fenomenología imaginaria de trabajar con un adulto joven

RESUMEN

Este artículo presenta una fenomenología imaginaria de trabajar con un adulto joven en psicoterapia. El caso indica la importancia de las "derivas' tácitas y/o inconscientes de significado y comunicación entre el cliente y el terapeuta. Como terapeutas podemos encontrar algo inesperado a través del cliente. Lo que surgen son aspectos de cómo explicamos/entendemos en retrospectiva, que se exploran brevemente a través de sentidos de diferencia, alienación, represión, ficción y muerte. Las racionalizaciones, y la conciencia de la experiencia, introducen algo muerto. Se explora la importancia de que el cliente hable por sí mismo. Los jóvenes especialmente parece necesitar encontrar su propio lenguaje de experiencia, sin ser aplastados por las palabras (y la presencia) de los demás, pero cómo esto suceda puede estar lleno de dificultad.

Che differenza fai, una fenomenologia immaginaria del lavoro con un giovane adulto

Questo articolo presenta una fenomenologia immaginaria del lavoro con un giovane adulto in psicoterapia. Il caso indica l'importanza di 'derapate' tacite e/o inconsce di significato e comunicazione tra cliente e terapeuta. Come terapeuti possiamo trovare qualcosa di inaspettato in noi stessi attraverso il cliente. Ne emerge come spieghiamo/comprendiamo in retrospettiva, che vengono brevemente esplorati attraverso i sensi di dissenso, alienazione, repressione, finzione e morte. Le razionalizzazioni e lo studio dell'esperienza introducono qualcosa di morto. Viene considerata l'importanza che il cliente utilizzi il suo linguaggio. Soprattutto i giovani sembrano aver bisogno di trovare un proprio linguaggio per narrare l'esperienza, senza essere schiacciati dalle parole (e dalla presenza) degli altri, tuttavia perseguire questo obiettivo sembra particolarmente irto di difficoltà.

Quel différend faites-vous ? Une phénoménologie imaginaire du travail avec un jeune adulte

Cet article présente une phénoménologie imaginaire du travail psychothérapeutique avec un jeune adulte. Ce cas pointe l'importance des « dérives » tacites et/ou inconscientes du sens et de la communication entre client et thérapeute. En tant que thérapeutes nous pourrions découvrir en nous ce qui est inattendu à travers le client. Émergent ainsi des aspects de la façon dont nous expliquons/comprenons rétrospectivement, aspects brièvement passés en revue à l'aide des notions de différend, d'aliénation, de refoulement, de fiction et de mort. Les rationalisations et la scientisation de l'expérience introduisent quelque chose de mortifère. L'importance pour un client de parler en son nom propre est abordée. Les jeunes plus particulièrement ont besoin de trouver leur propre langage d'expérience sans risquer d'être écrasés par les mots (et la présence) des autres. Que ce soit possible reste un parcours semé d'embuches.

Τι διαφορά κάνεις. Μια φανταστική φαινομενολογία της συνεργασίας με έναν νεαρό ενήλικα

ΠΕΡΊΛΗΨΗ

Αυτό το άρθρο παρουσιάζει μια φανταστική φαινομενολογία της συνεργασίας με έναν νεαρό ενήλικα στην ψυχοθεραπεία. Η περίπτωση δείχνει τη σημασία της σιωπηρής και/ή ασυνείδητης «μετατόπισης» του νοήματος και της επικοινωνίας μεταξύ πελάτη και θεραπευτή. Ως θεραπευτές μπορεί να συναντήσουμε αυτό που ήταν απροσδόκητο σε εμάς στον πελάτη μας. Αυτό που αναδύεται είναι πτυχές του τρόπου με τον οποίο εξηγούμε/αντιλαμβανόμαστε αναδρομικά, οι οποίες διερευνώνται εν συντομία μέσα από τις αισθήσεις της διαφοροποίησης, της αποξένωσης, της καταστολής, της μυθοπλασίας και του θανάτου. Ο εξορθολογισμός και η επιστημονικοποίηση της εμπειρίας εισάγουν κάτι νεκρό. Διερευνάται η σημασία του να μιλάει ο πελάτης για τον εαυτό του. Οι νέοι ειδικά, φαίνεται ότι πρέπει να βρουν τη δική τους βιωματική γλώσσα, χωρίς να συνθλίβονται από τις λέξεις (και την παρουσία) των άλλων, αλλά το πώς αυτό είναι δυνατό μοιάζει δύσκολο.

SCHLÜSSELWÖRTER Unterschied; Phänomenologie; Fall vignette; junger Erwachsener; Psychotherapie; Fiktion

PALABRAS CLAVE diferencia; fenomenología; caso de estudio; adulto joven; psicoterapia; ficción

PAROLE CHIAVE dissenso; fenomenologia; case study; giovani adulti; psicoterapia; finzione

MOTS-CLÉS différend; phénoménologie; étude de cas; jeune adulte; psychothérapie; fiction

ΛΈΞΕΙΣ ΚΛΕΙΔΙΆ διαφοροποίηση; φαινομενολογία; μελέτη περίπτωσης; νεαρός ενήλικας; ψυχοθεραπεία; μυθοπλασία

Introduction

What is in play in this imaginary case study (Part 2) is largely tacit, in that it is likely that the reader will read his/her own meanings into what is presented. Some aspects which the narrative invoked in the author's mind *in retrospect* (Part 1) have to do with differend, meta-language, experience, repression, alienation, fiction/non-fiction, and death. The approach to presenting these aspects and the narrative of the case is considered to be phenomenological, in that what is placed before us, in our thinking, our bodies, and in our relation to the world – what is 'within' us – is taken seriously, or noticed (as opposed to being theorised or rationalised). In Merleau-Ponty's words,

> The relation to the world, such as it tirelessly announces itself within us, is not something that analysis might clarify: philosophy can simply place it before our eyes and invite us to take notice (Merleau- Ponty, 1945/2014, pp. xxxii/18).

In terms of being psychotherapeutic, this 'noticing' may help us come to see the ways in which we do not hear/see our clients, entwined as we are in our own 'ideologies' of our training, our personal history, and experiences of living. Do we notice the effects on the therapy of the intertwining of *our own* experience of being a person, and once (or perhaps still, at many levels) a young adult? To quote an icon of anxious young adults from the 1980s, Morrisey (*The Smiths*), 'What difference does it make?' (Marr & Morrissey, 1984).

Part 1

Differend, meta-language, experience, and repression

'Differend' is a word the young adult in this imaginary case study would have liked. Lyotard (1988) invented it to describe the phenomenon of say, A's attempting to communicate being elided through the 'translation' of that communication into another's, say B's language, meaning, and experience. It is as if A's experience is passed through a filter of the other's language, that of B's, such that A's experience no longer exists, even as if it never existed. This traumatic experience happens all the time. B has the power here. Here is a personal example, necessarily fictionalised. I (A) was once accused by a supervisor (B) of coming to a supervision session drunk. I was so nonplussed by the accusation, or rather, the supposedly therapeutically delivered suggestion, that I sat in silence in complete bewilderment. The suggestion was so off the mark that the effect was to block something out. After a few long seconds of blankness something kicked back to life and I understood suddenly then that my Irish accent, with its drawl and way of running words together, its foreignness, my slightly flushed face from caffeine, and anxiety at seeing this new supervisor (as he had forgotten about our previous appointment), was what he was 'interpreting' with that certainty of the professional ideologue. Without knowing such a word existed, I certainly felt I was subject to 'differend', and anything I said would be interpreted as a denial of some kind. I nervously informed him that he was mistaken. He seemed satisfied and reassured that I was lying. I was lying, of course, but not in the way he thought. The supervision session continued on formal guidelines then, I paid the fee, and never went back. Somehow even to enter into any dialogue on the subject of his error would have only confirmed more his view that he was correct. There was no place for my words to find a hearing. The poor supervisor's certainty would have been pathetic if it had not been so offensive and professionally dangerous. This was perhaps a shade of a Brexit moment in its worst form – the 'foreign other' receives all the projections that deep-rooted myth, fiction, and cultural lies can muster.

A different way of thinking of 'differend' is to consider how there is no such thing as a meta-language (Lacan, 1977, p. 311). It is easy to get caught up in Lacan's thought, its mesmeric power, like staring into a wild river and not realising you have already fallen in. Nevertheless, it seems so true that we cannot find a language that can speak adequately of the 'truth' of being, that gets 'above being'.

> No language can speak the truth about truth, since truth establishes herself by speaking, and by having no other means to do so (Lacan, 1966, pp. 867-868).

As Borch-Jacobsen (1991, p. 110) elaborates, truth 'speaks herself mischievously – fictionally, mythically – ... '. We can just speak, invent, and stumble along. There is no language that speaks of language from 'above' language. Whenever we do attempt to do this, there is an imposition – an exercise of power that some authority announces – that guarantees validity. We define parameters in order to contain what meanings are allowed, but something always falls outside of those. There is a sense here of the difference between language and speaking. Speech tends to show how words themselves have 'hooked into' our very flesh. We may notice this in therapy when a client stumbles over an everyday word. They have found something that has a unique significance to them, that no pre-defined 'catalogue of meanings' could have predicted or known. We can come to speak our own truth, but we cannot impose that on another person as if it is their truth, as if in a language of 'universal truth' (a meta-language).

It seems that the founder of phenomenology, Husserl, too was looking for a meta-language of sorts, a foundation of all sciences based on the limitations of consciousness. Husserl's phenomenology could be said to be a rejection of a 'realistic and naturalistic objectivism' that claims that the nature of meaning, truth and reality can be understood without taking subjectivity into account (Zahavi, 2003, p. 52). Husserl is touching on something that is similar to Lyotard and Lacan, in that one's subjectivity does something to meaning that we cannot get away from. Husserl's concept of a kind of anonymous pre-reflective self-awareness (Husserl, 1997, p. 478; Zahavi, 2003, p. 92) functioning in our everyday lives and experiences perhaps indicates that we 'do' something in relation that we cannot know about. It appears that it is a kind of 'false' experience that gathers experience as if it were 'above' experience (objective). To take off the spectacles of presumption in psychotherapy; to take out the function of 'predictive texting' in our language (eg in being certain we know best for our client), we open up our senses to that world announcing itself in the intertwining of language and experience. We are already immersed in language and experience as we attempt to communicate always within that immersion. After a neatly presented talk, for example, no matter how 'evidence-based', or even 'grounded in reality', surely, we must know we've been fooling ourselves. Our carefully prepared 'talk' is dislocated from our 'being.' Husserl's failure to find the ground of consciousness, after a life's work (Zahavi, 2003), perhaps poignantly indicates this immersion. He did not see, until much later in his life perhaps (Zahavi, 2003), what Heidegger (1993, p. 217) saw, that 'language is the house of Being'.

Alienation

There is the real sense that our words bend into a rigidity, forming thoughts and lines of thinking that seem impossible to break out from, or to even think the thought that such a 'breaking out' is possible. It does seem that we are 'forced' into language, 'alienated' in its meanings and structures. The cage of language can also be a safe place to be. Perhaps being alienated from this alienation is what allows madness and poetry. One way of 'seeing' this alienation is to watch an old film. The ways of expression seem 'natural' to the protagonists but looking back from our distance of many years, we can see how language has channelled, shaped, or 'cut into' their experience. Something is suppressed or even repressed. Language bends our thought like the light bends a stick in water.

An example from Freud (Forrester, 1997, pp. 13–15) perhaps shows one way in which language distorts something. The story is of King Solomon deciding how to judge the case of two women arguing over a baby. Each woman had her own baby and they shared a home together, but during the night one woman rolled onto her baby and it died. She then swapped her dead baby for the living one. Before Solomon, the women are each claiming the surviving baby is her own. King Solomon orders that the living child can be shared but divided in two by sword. The story continues, with one of the women speaking out.

> "I beg you, my lord,' she said, 'let them give her the live child; on no account let them kill him!' But the other said, 'He shall belong to neither of us. Cut him in half!' Then the king gave his decision, 'Give the live child to the first woman,' he said, 'and do not kill him. She is his mother.' (1 Kings: 26-28 in *New Jerusalem Bible* (1990)).

We are struck by the wisdom of Solomon, and the love of the true mother. But Forrester (1997) notes the impact on our awareness on reading Freud's (1921/2001, pp. 120–121) comments on this story regarding social justice, ' ... the same germ is to be found in the apt story of the judgement of Solomon. If one woman's child is dead, the other shall not have a live one either. The bereaved woman is recognised by this wish.'

Freud's comment shows how we have been 'led away' by the narrative of the Biblical story (Forrester, 1997, p. 15). We see the goodness of a mother, rather than the lethal envy of a mother, in a way that almost seems we have repressed the latter. Perhaps most of us would not want to know about this form that envy can take and its consequences. Freud (1921/2001) drily notes, 'Social justice means that we deny ourselves many things so that others may have to do without them as well' (see Forrester, 1997, p. 15).

Death and the word

When we speak presuming (tacitly or otherwise) we are in a metalanguage, it is like we are speaking from an ideology, and it feels as if death has entered into the words. The words require the precision of a legal document and they indeed become the death of something. It can be seen how in a negative sense, a non-therapeutic sense, 'the letter kills ... ' (Lacan, 2006, p. 719). Rather than protecting us from an overwhelming experience – which would be in theory therapeutic, the talking cure (Fink, 1995, p. 25) – instead the word kills off something. It seems that in most of the psychological sciences now words are used tacitly in that negative sense so that experience is killed. Experience is either rationalised or put through the filter of scientism. There is no curiosity, or wondering about, for example, as to the form language is forming. Experience becomes replaced by an ideology of knowledge. A sleight of hand happens – or what is really an assumption so all-encompassing that we do not notice it – so that in this ideology we cannot say we know anything without tacitly referring to its terms of reference. We are like bees inside a jam jar living on sugared water not knowing the whole wider world of experience is outside the glass. We think we are already outside the glass. It is possible that the young sense this more than the old but having no words of their own to guide them perhaps this is why some attempt to cut their way out. How often have we heard a young person saying to us therapists, professional listeners, 'No, you're not listening.' A young client once found the courage to shout at me for 'silencing' her with ideas. She was (almost completely) right, and I apologised. In the long silences that followed over the following weeks, forgiveness somehow found its way back into the space between us. A book or two could be written about what must have happened in the silences of those sessions.

Fiction/non-fiction

The case study presented here is fictional. The insecurity, the enthusiasm, the ability to trust in a burgeoning bodily experience of life on the client's part; the envy, regret and sadness on the therapist's part. These are just some threads running through its fabric. If it can be useful for those working in non-fictional counselling and psychotherapy sessions, then perhaps it will serve a purpose. But this raises the question of fiction in all psychological therapies generally. To perhaps think that our own narratives, familial and cultural stories, fantasies, our 'clear thinking', do not intertwine with those of our clients is possibly a fiction in itself. So, it seems that it is not so much the content of this fictional case study that is important but rather sensitivity to the insight that emerges *in retrospect*, even in retrospect seconds after we have said something 'insightful.' We are affected by the other, and our own stories in a way that we do not understand in advance, it seems, and how those effects affect or grip us will determine everything.

So what difference does it make?

Some of the significance of the difference all this makes can perhaps be read between the lines of this account – or even read unconsciously, 'not consciously known' (*unbewusst*) (Strachey, 1957/2001, p. 165). The account of this imaginary case was mainly driven by unknown intuitive 'decisions' Which we then stick meaning to after the fact. But it is as if these 'intuitive moves' indicate something of a landscape extending underground, something beneath a topography. The words of the young Sigmund Freud's mentor, Ewald Hering, come to mind:

> Who could hope to disentangle the fabric of our inner life with its thousand-fold complexities, if we were willing to pursue its threads only so far as they traverse consciousness? ... ... For the mind would often slip through the fingers of psychology, if psychology refused to keep a hold on the mind's unconscious states (Hering, 1870, pp. 11;13 in Strachey, 1957/2001, p. 205).

Whether we can 'keep a hold' on unconscious states seems unlikely, but it is possible to pay attention, to wait, to allow what may come to mind come to mind and not turn away. This staying with experience, just as we might stay with a dream, is a phenomenological stance (Zahavi, 2003). The phenomenological here just describes the landscape but does not pretend to be disinterested as a scientific method would. This *disinterest/interest* makes a difference, as to how we listen. Freud's term, *Bezetsung*, is significant here, translated by Strachey into the technical *cathexis*, but surely much more apposite in its original, more ordinary meaning as 'interest' (Gay, 1995, p. 89). Our 'interest' (and 'disinterest') nudges us along, not necessarily in the best directions. For example, can we bear to explore properly why we may have an interest in one client and not another?

The problem with technique seems to be the same as the problem with the certainty of our disinterest/interest, or any words used too often so that we assume we know what they mean, in that they accumulate an inertia around them, acting like strings of gravity from which nothing escapes. They make cuts and ruts in the fabric of the mind along which ideologies are drawn. They accumulate into ropes that bind us, rein us in, without knowing much about it. Ordinary words, those ones that lie around like 'rubbish' paperback novels, or 'rubbish' songs, instead don't bind but cut, their edges like little knives that cut through the gravity inertia rut rope, splaying apart its fibres to show its colours, forms, and arguments.

The phenomenological described here simply uses those words that are at hand to describe the world 'tirelessly announcing itself'. What seems most important is that we catch ourselves weaving ropes of thought that bind us, and others, and wonder about that. Perhaps there is importance in binding thoughts sometimes.

Part 2

This is the case (it reads better if you read it out loud while walking around)

We chose you because you're so well qualified. Mother's eyes boring in. Trying to fish out a nod of collusion from my blank look she must catch as a dumb stare. He's an adult not a child. And so am I. It's confidential. We understand you can't give us feedback. Good. But they're paying. I should insist that the young man pays, but later I see that this tack is hopeless. He has no money. It would be a sham to pretend he was paying. The mother wants to come in too, but some slight shift in me gets the message across that that wouldn't be the right thing to do, so she smiles grimly and leaves.

I show him to the room and he takes his place slightly dazed in look at first, looking around like a large animal worried and out of its natural habitat. He says he hasn't been out of the house in weeks. He likes playing computer games with his mates online. The Lacanian in me ticking boxes – I make the effort to close the door rudely on Lacan in his lecture theatre in my head, much to his annoyance, and I try to be more phenomenological. Phenomenology is just about noticing what is there before your eyes, or your senses. What belongs to whom, and what seems co-produced between us, and why would that be. And it's also about getting out of the way of your client, to let them come forward, and noticing in that trying to get out of the way, what things seem to belong to both of us. I thought I had discovered for myself how Husserl's (1970) phenomenological reduction – the putting aside of our assumptions about a phenomenon – could be seen as just this 'getting out of the way' of the other (McSherry, 2018), but accidentally found the same phrase in a musician's work recently:

> The most, the best, we can do, we/believe (wanting to give evidence of/love), is to get out of the way, leave/space around whomever or whatever it is (Cage, 1967 cited in Nelson, 2012).

I don't say any of this, of course, but it flees across my mind like a small animal taking cover behind the books as I sit down.

He hesitantly talks about computer games and friends as his main interests. But he is scanning my face and room, my clothes and look, like a master craftsman getting the measure of something. I will have to fight for some purchase, as it seems like I have already been dismissed, condemned by some quirk he must have noticed, or by the books on my shelves. I can't help but like this strange creature. How often do we look in the mirror and ask ourselves who is that strange creature staring back? A wild thought crosses my mind that I want to set him free. He says his parents thought it was a good idea for him to come and talk to someone, and he thinks it would be good as well. I wonder.

His parents' plans – or rather his mother and his stepfather's plans, as he never met his father – their plans for his life are different to his. He doesn't have any. They're paying for the therapy. They want results. Back to university and get a girlfriend. He thinks girls are pointless – they only want one thing.

Love.
It's too much.
They're scary.

They're nice sometimes but scary. They're as nasty as boys, in a different way. And it all seems a bit pointless. I get an image of a smooth road mapped out before him, bland as a pancake with no syrup, honey, butter, or lemon. The future that invites him is labelled – 'wasteland.' No wonder he takes flight into the virtual world of computer games. It's better than the real thing.

I should find a nice girl and get married. I know that. I could get a job. My father knows people. He's talking like he already knows I think these same thoughts as his parents' thoughts. I'm in their age group. I think of my own life at 20. Full of the need to be accepted into the world of others and being accepted sexually. Society and love occupied me. Is that bit about love too feminine? He thinks love is for girls. Is that why it seems he has dismissed me? Or is the feeling something to do with him, with both of us perhaps? I will dismiss his thoughts like his parents do, so he's dismissing me first. There's more to it than that. That's just a glimpse of a wider unknown landscape between us which perhaps both of us share.

His body was too big for his mind. Although he came out with sparky genius sentences – how on earth had he read anything of Levinas at his age? – it seemed his mind was still forming, trying to crystallise onto some ideology to guide him. Looking for a master signifier to latch onto besides the tired old clichés his parents were pressing on him. Yes, he knew Freud too, but he was just another doctor. And clearly mad. Oh. Or a pervert. And Levinas was just soft. Just a softy. He's like our vicar. Christ. I don't mean to insult you, my mother said you liked Freud. It said it on your website. But he charged too much for his sessions. He only saw rich people, didn't he?

A dim envy occupied me, of a mind just forming that could drop Freud with such carefree dash. That could face down Levinas. Dismissing the professors with a shrug of an almost teenage shoulder, skittering past the old fogies doing a wheelie on his mountain bike. You don't need therapy I want to blurt out – *but your parents do*. You just need to go and live. Just go and live! Go and make your own mistakes rather than the mistakes of others. Come back in ten years if it's all getting a bit too much. But for some reason I don't say that. I do the therapist thing and encourage him to speak, to say what is on his mind. I fit into the role it seems already prepared for me by his parents and I listen benevolently like a concerned uncle. Not quite one of the family. Some things about his body that embarrass him. Not to worry. Give yourself some time. He accepted my reassurance simply, in contrast to everything else – disarmingly respectful.

After that first session I got an email from his mother saying she thought her son had benefited from our meeting, and already looked better. They wanted to book another session for the following week. They would make sure he got there. I felt pleased. The young adult in me felt pleased that his parents had been pleased. But approval would be measured out week by week depending on something. On what? The confusion of who to please, and what should be pleasing, had already infected the relationships like a virus. Needing a firewall, I replied curtly and confirmed the next appointment. This young man's trouble was his parents. And if I didn't watch it, my parents would become his trouble too. A troubling sentence formed itself in the air somewhere, saying something like 'if you fit in with what we want, things will go well, but if not, well, we'll see … '

In a world that is difficult, where education counts, where being unemployed for too long may lead to a slippery slope into depression and misery, how could I not have sympathy for his parents? But surely my job was to open up a space for him to hear his own thoughts and appreciate those, no matter what thoughts may come. In standing as an opposing force to his parents, while also wanting to please them, was I not contradicting myself? He would know soon enough if I were colluding with them in order to please, and in order to be paid also. But I wouldn't fall in to such a simple trap. My worry was more how much I was *already* like his parents, so that I would be *already* nudging him towards the bland horizon without even knowing it. I tried to watch out for any slight nod in that direction coming from me, any slight smile, grimace, movement of my legs or hands, anything at all that seemed to push him towards something.

The next session. He said everything went well over the last week. Far less computer time. And more thinking about getting into university. He had the ability, he knew, but it was a matter of knowing what to do. He wanted to do computer gaming as a career. A game designer and tester. I flinched. It sounded horrific to me, stuck in front of computers all day, but I nodded acceptingly. His mother wanted him to do law. Inwardly, I thought that law sounded good but outwardly I said nothing.

I fall into line in my thoughts, treading an awkward place between his desires and pragmatism, what I would like him to do if he were my child, and what I would do if I were him. I imagined I would have liked to have had a mother who exerted such ambitious and practical demands on me. Law would be good. Better than gaming maybe. But it was up to him. Weeks pass. The physical problems no longer worry him so much. It was helpful to talk to someone with a science background about that. His young vulnerability doesn't admit that it was nice just to have someone benevolent to speak to about it. I hadn't done science in 30 years.

Then one day he comes in and gives me a kindly lecture. I can see he has come to trust me somehow. He can see that therapy has a place. It's important. Freud was good. But Lacan is better. It's a pity we haven't spoken more about Lacan as he sees I have some books about him on my shelves. And Wittgenstein too. He was a character. Gave all his money away to live more freely. What about that book of poems by Heaney, maybe we could have read some of those? He was always talking about mud, bogs and frogspawn though. But all this stuff and all this therapy is not the same as living. He just has to 'go and live' doesn't he? I nod mutely, smiling inwardly, confused and caught out in some way I don't yet understand. He had caught the drift of my drift (Freud, 1923/2001, p. 239), despite myself, and was following where I wished he would go all along from the very start. How could I ever know that this was what he wanted, or was it just what he thought I wanted from him (another substitute parent to please)? How can we ever know? I thought of Lacan's (2006, pp. 21/30) words about everything following the path of the signifier – '. . . destiny, refusals, blindnesses, success and fate . . . '. Opening a door to that lecture theatre in my head he was standing there, waving a harsh finger at me. Was my client following some instruction to please the other?

> I just have to live.
> Yes, I said, just go swimming in life. Try it out.

He fleetingly looked apprehensive, a young boy for the first time walking to school on his own.

And drop back to see me whenever you want, I reassure him. I'm here. I'm not going anywhere as far as I know. I hoped he would drop back some day for my own sake too. I would feel lonely without this awkward genius disturbing my worried mind.

He left that day and I never saw him again. I imagined him vaulting over the gate, or maybe crashing through it, and doing wheelies down the footpath home. For a moment I wished I was his age again, knowing nothing, yet enough to crash through gates. After he left, I write my notes like an obsessive religious scraping out an epitaph. I realise I'd forgotten to ask him what his plans were. They mustn't have been that important.

I got no more emails from his mother, and the final payment was withheld.

Youth had caught me out, outshone and outstripped me, as it should do. I was needed just to hold a space for him for a while, keep him safe enough to hear his own words, catch his own drift and go with that. There would be time enough for him to realise if it were someone else's drift he had caught, mistaking it for his own. He could be trusted to right his own errors and find his own way. He left me with some kind of drift also, that didn't seem to be mine, or found a home in me that was already prepared. I didn't know what. Until much later, tears of grief came. Of course – or is it that obvious? – I was recalling my own dark-haired young self, the insecurity of it all, but flying in the face of that insecurity somehow too. And my father anxiously asking me to get a good job with a pension. There is much more, of course, that could be written.

In place of a discussion and conclusion

For the bewildered listener/reader, the young scientist can summarise something. Firstly, the temptation to collude with the authorities is great, and with one's own authorities (for example, Lacan). Even in trying not to do this, by whose authority do we try not to do it, and have we scrutinised that authority (under whose authority, and so on)? Another way of putting this is to ask what differend is in play if we try to take out of play any differend? Secondly, an answer to this last question might be in the thought of how being neutral as the therapist seems mistaken. And in the place of neutrality can we place an oscillating uncertainty, a willingness to be completely wrong? It seems impossible to be present without imparting something of one's own ideology. Thirdly, what seems so clear is the importance of being present, secure in one's presence, like the edge of a riverbank needed as something to kick off from. We are needed to stay in place so the other can push away from us. We neither give way, nor hold, nor follow. At least none of these too much. The loneliness of working with someone much younger in this case, is in this holding still and letting go. There is a grief here and acceptance of it.

Finally, in all of this the ideology I seemed to be imparting was 'you are able to find your own way, you were built for it'; which I believe is to paraphrase some of Seamus Heaney's (1998, p. 231) words,

> "Before the kite plunges down into the wood,
> and this line goes useless,
> take in your two hands, boys, and feel
> The strumming, rooted, long-tailed pull of grief.
> You were born fit for it.

Stand in here in front of me
and take the strain."

(*A Kite for Michael and Christopher*)

Disclosure statement

No potential conflict of interest was reported by the author(s).

References

Borch-Jacobsen, M. (1991). *Lacan: The absolute master*. D. Brick, trans. Stanford University Press.

Cage, J. (1967). *A Year from Monday: New Lectures and Writings*. Wesleyan University Press.

Fink, B. (1995). *The Lacanian subject - Between language and jouissance*. Princeton University Press.

Forrester, J. (1997). *Dispatches from the Freud Wars: Psychoanalysis and its passions*. Harvard University Press.

Freud, S. (1921/2001). Group psychology and the analysis of the ego. In J. Strachey (Ed.), *The standard edition of the complete psychoanalytical works of Sigmund Freud* (Vol. XVIII, pp. 235–259). Vintage, The Hogarth Press and The Institute of Psychoanalysis.

Freud, S. (1923/2001). Two encyclopaedia articles. In J. Strachey (Ed.), *The standard edition of the complete psychoanalytical works of Sigmund Freud* (Vol. XVIII, pp. 120–121). Vintage, The Hogarth Press and The Institute of Psychoanalysis.

Gay, P. (1995). *The Freud reader*. Vintage.

Heaney, S. (1998). *Opened ground: Poems 1966-1996*. Faber and Faber.

Heidegger, M. (1993). *Basic writings* (2nd ed.) (D. F. Krell (Ed.)). Harper- San Francisco.

Hering, E. (1870). *Über das Gedächtnisä als eine allgemeine Function der organisirten Materie*. Lecture to the Imperial Academy of Sciences, Vienna, May 30. Published as pamphlet.

Husserl, E. (1970). *The crisis of European sciences and transcendental phenomenology: An introduction to phenomenological philosophy* (D. Carr, Trans.). Northwestern University Press.

Husserl, E. (1997). *Psychological and transcendental phenomenology and the confrontation with Heidegger*. T. Sheehan and R. E. Palmer (Eds.), (Thomas Sheehan and Richard E. Palmer, Trans.). Kluwer Academic Publishers.

Lacan, J. (1966). *Écrits*. Seiul: Paris.

Lacan, J. (1977). *Écrits: A selection*. (A. Sheridan, Trans.). Norton.

Lacan, J. (2006). *Écrits, the first complete edition in English*. (B. Fink, H. Fink, & R. Grigg, Trans.). W. W. Norton & Co.

Lyotard, J. (1988). *The differend: Phrases in dispute*. (G. Van Den Abeele, Trans.). University of Minnesota Press.

Marr, J., & Morrissey, S. (1984). What difference does it make? Lyrics. (n.d.) *Lyrics. com*. Retrieved February 4, 2020, from http://www.lyrics.com/lyric/4545619/Face +to+Face

McSherry, A. (2018). *What is the need, if any, for therapeutic education in mental health nursing? An empirical phenomenological study of mental health nurses' responses to this question* [Unpublished PhD thesis]. Research Centre for Therapeutic Education, Dept. of Psychology, Roehampton University.

Merleau- Ponty, M. (1945/2014). *Phenomenology of perception*. (D. A. Landes, Trans.). Routledge.

Nelson, M. (2012). *The art of cruelty: A Reckoning*. W. W. Norton & Co.

Strachey, J. (1957/2001a). Editor's note. In J. Strachey (Ed.), *The standard edition of the complete psychoanalytical works of Sigmund Freud* (Vol. XIV, p. 165). Vintage, The Hogarth Press and The Institute of Psychoanalysis.

Strachey, J. (1957/2001b). Appendix A: Freud and Ewald Hering. In J. Strachey (Ed.), *The standard edition of the complete psychoanalytical works of Sigmund Freud* (Vol. XIV, p. 205). Vintage, The Hogarth Press and The Institute of Psychoanalysis.

Zahavi, D. (2003). *Husserl's phenomenology*. Stanford University Press.

Finishing school, fishing and flourishing: Appetite, engagement and compliance in Daoism, Existentialism and Psychoanalysis

Onel Brooks

ABSTRACT

After an account of working as a psychotherapist, some affinities, similarities and intersections between Zhuangzi, Nietzsche and Heidegger and some versions of psychoanalysis are identified. These include warnings about our overvaluation of calculative knowledge, our equating thinking with rational, calculative thinking, and our being dominated by a technological view of all things, including ourselves. The writers drawn together here emphasise vastness, complexity, ambiguity, contrasting this with our smallness, finitude, our limitedness, our tendency to conform, comply and crave certainty. In contrast to technological thinking and convictions, they favour and show a kind of indirectness, meandering, a freedom to associate and wander, the cultivation of a capacity to take a view that is less constrained. They value our capacity to be solitary, to be ourself, and they are at least suspicious of the desire to be like everyone else. They champion being able to face pain and suffering without losing our love and appetite for life.

Abschluss der Schule, Fischen und Blühen Appetit, Engagement und Compliance in Daoismus, Existenzialismus und Psychoanalyse

ABSTRACT

Nach einem Bericht über die Arbeit als Psychotherapeut werden einige Affinitäten, Ähnlichkeiten und Überschneidungen zwischen Zhuangzi, Nietzsche und Heidegger sowie einige Versionen der Psychoanalyse identifiziert. Dazu gehören Warnungen vor unserer Überbewertung des rechnerischen Wissens, unserem Gleichsetzen des Denkens mit rationalem, rechnerischem Denken und unserer Dominanz durch eine technologische Sicht auf alle Dinge, einschließlich uns selbst. Die hier zusammengestellten Autoren betonen Weite, Komplexität, Mehrdeutigkeit und kontrastieren dies mit unserer Kleinheit, Endlichkeit, unserer Begrenztheit, unserer Tendenz, sich anzupassen, zu entsprechen und nach Gewissheit zu verlangen. Im Gegensatz zu technologischem Denken und Überzeugungen bevorzugen und zeigen sie eine Art von Indirektheit, Mäandern, Freiheit zu assoziieren und zu wandern, die Kultivierung einer Fähigkeit, eine weniger eingeschränkte Sichtweise zu vertreten. Sie schätzen unsere Fähigkeit, einsam zu sein, wir selbst zu sein, und sie sind zumindest misstrauisch gegenüber dem Wunsch, wie alle anderen zu sein. Sie setzen sich dafür ein, Schmerzen und Leiden begegnen zu können, ohne unsere Liebe und unseren Appetit auf das Leben zu verlieren.

Terminar la escuela, pescar, florecer Apetito, compromiso y cumplimiento en el Daoísmo, Existencialismo y Psicoanálisis

RESUMEN

Después de un relato trabajando como psicoterapeuta, se pueden dentificar algunas similitudes e intersecciones afines entre Zhuangzi, Nietzsche y Heidegger y algunas versiones del psicoanálisis. Estas incluyen advertencias sobre nuestra sobrevaloración del conocimiento calculativo, nuestro pensamiento equiparado con el pensamiento racional y calculativo, y nuestro ser dominado por una visión tecnológica de todas las cosas, incluyéndonos a nosotros mismos. Los escritores reunidos aquí enfatizan la inmensidad, la complejidad, la ambiguedad, contrastando esto con nuestra pequeidad, finitud, nuestra limitación, nuestra tendencia a conformarse, cumplir y anhelar la certeza. En contraste con el pensamiento tecnológico y las convicciones, favorecen y muestran una especie de indirecto, serpenteante, libertad de asociación y deambulamiento, el cultivo de una capacidad para tomar una visión menos limitada. Valoran nuestra capacidad de ser solitarios, de ser nosotros mismos, y al menos dudan del deseo de ser como todos los demás. Abogan por enfrentar el dolor y el sufrimiento sin perder nuestro amor y el interés por la vida.

Scuola di perfezionamento, Appetito fiorente, impegno e rispetto nel Daoismo, nell'Esistenzialismo e in Psicoanalisi

Dopo aver narrato l'espereinza come psicoterapeuta, vengono identificate alcune affinità, somiglianze e intersezioni tra Zhuangzi, Nietzsche e Heidegger e alcune versioni della psicoanalisi. Ciò include raccomandazioni sulla nostra tendenza a sopravvalutare la conoscenza calcolativa, il nostro pensiero razionale e il nostro essere dominati da una visione tecnologica di tutte le cose, incluso noi stessi. Gli autori, posti a confronto, sottolineano la vastità, la complessità, l'ambiguità e le confrontano con la umana piccolezza, finitudine, la nostra limitatezza, la nostra tendenza a conformarci, rispettare e desiderare la certezza. Contrariamente al pensiero tecnologico e alle convinzioni certe, incoraggiano una sorta di posizione indiretta, meandri, libertà di associazione e di distrazione, dedicarsi alla capacità di avere una visione meno vincolata. È inoltre sostenuta la capacità di stare in solitudine, di essere se stessi, mentre è visto con sospetto il desiderio di essere come tutti gli altri. In tal modo si è in grado di affrontare il dolore e la sofferenza senza perdere l'amore e l'*appetito* per la vita.

La fin de l'école, la pêche et un appétit grandissant: engagement et respect des règles dans le taoïsme, l'existentialisme et la psychanalyse

Après la description de mon travail en tant que psychothérapeute, j'identifie des affinités, similarités et intersections entre Zhuangzi, Nietzsche et Heidegger et certaines versions de la psychanalyse. Cela inclut des avertissements sur notre surévaluation du savoir calculé, notre façon d'équivaloir la pensée à la pensée rationnelle et calculée et notre domination par une vue technologique de toutes choses y compris de nous-mêmes. Les auteurs auxquels nous faisons référence ici mettent l'accent sur la vastitude, la complexité, l'ambiguïté contrastant avec notre petitesse, notre finitude, nos limitations, notre tendance à nous conformer, à obéir et notre besoin de certitude. À la pensée et aux convictions technologiques, ils préfèrent et prennent des détours, des méandres, associent librement et s'égarent tout en cultivant une capacité à adopter un point de vue moins étriqué. Ils valorisent notre capacité à la solitude, à être soi-même et sont suspicieux quant au désir d'être comme tout le monde. Ils soutiennent avec ardeur la capacité à faire face à la douleur et à la souffrance sans pour autant perdre notre amour et notre appétit pour la vie.

Τελειώνοντας το σχολείο, βρίσκοντας και καλλιεργώντας την όρεξη, δέσμευση και συμμόρφωση στον Ταοϊσμό, τον Υπαρξισμό και την Ψυχανάλυση

ΠΕΡΊΛΗΨΗ:

Μετά την εμπειρία εργασίας ως ψυχοθεραπευτής, εντοπίζονται ορισμένες συγγένειες, ομοιότητες και διασταυρώσεις μεταξύ των Zhuangzi, Nietzsche και Heidegger και με ορισμένες εκδοχές της ψυχανάλυσης. Αυτές αποτελούν προειδοποιήσεις σχετικά με την υπερεκτίμηση της υπολογιστικής γνώσης, την εξίσωση της σκέψης μας με την λογική, την υπολογιστική σκέψη και την κυριαρχία μας από μια τεχνολογική θέαση όλων των πραγμάτων, συμπεριλαμβανομένου και του εαυτού μας. Οι συγγραφείς που συγκεντρώνονται εδώ τονίζουν την απεραντοσύνη, την πολυπλοκότητα, την ασάφεια, που αντιπαρέχονται του μικρού μας μέγεθος, των περιορισμών, των ορίων μας, της τάσης μας για συμμόρφωση, συμφωνία και λαχτάρα για βεβαιότητα. Σε αντίθεση με την τεχνολογική σκέψη και τις πεποιθήσεις, ευνοούν και δείχνουν ένα είδος έμμεσου και άσκοπου, μια ελευθερία για σύνδεση και περιπλάνηση, την καλλιέργεια μιας ικανότητας να λαμβάνει κανείς μια άποψη που είναι λιγότερο περιορισμένη. Εκτιμούν την ικανότητά μας να είμαστε μοναχικοί, να είμαστε ο εαυτός μας, και είναι τουλάχιστον καχύποπτοι για την επιθυμία του να είναι κανείς ίδιος με τους άλλους. Υποστηρίζουν την δυνατότητά μας για την αντιμετώπιση του πόνου και της ταλαιπωρίας, χωρίς να χάνουμε την αγάπη και την όρεξή μας για ζωή.

Schlüsselwörter Zhuangzi; Nietzsche; Heidegger; Freud; Winnicott; Phillips

PALABRAS CLAVE Zhuangzi; nietzsche; heidegger; freud; winnicott; phillips

MOTS-CLÉS Zhuangzi; Nietzsche; Heidegger; Freud; Winnicott; Phillips

Λέξεις κλειδιά Zhuangzi; Nietzsche; Heidegger; Freud; Winnicott; Phillips

'Saying is not blowing breath, saying says something: the only trouble is that what it says is never fixed. Do we really say something? Or have we never said anything?' (Zhuangzi chapter 3 in 1989, p. 52)

'Suppose I put it to you in abandoned words, and you listen with the same abandon ... ' (Zhuangzi chapter 3 in 1989, p. 59)

Introduction: Mastering, making, owning

A number of works discuss how Nietzsche and Heidegger are related to eastern philosophy and practices (for example, Cooper, 2014, 2018; Froese, 2006; Parkes, 1996). This is an attempt by a practitioner who has an appetite for existentialism and psychoanalysis to say something about how early or philosophical Daoism seems to anticipate important themes in Nietzsche, Heidegger and psychoanalysis, and may have much to interest, charm and provoke those who are concerned with psychotherapy.

Mesmerised by measuring, equating numbering with knowing, we might insist that everything and everyone must be stood up straight, made to salute, and get to the point, and that failure to do this should be thought about as evidence of 'oppositional defiant disorder', 'ODD' rather than 'exuberance'. In Zhuangzi, Nietzsche and some versions of psychoanalysis, there is a consensus of suspicion and opposition to the desire for consensus, clear conclusions and outcomes. The twists, turns, quirks and apparent dead ends are valued, paradoxes, parables and puzzles proliferate and are preferred to pointing out what is proper and perfect. There is acknowledgement that our 'knowing' is like standing on a familiar island in an ocean of what is unknown and perhaps unknowable.

Chuang-Tzu, Chuang Chou, Zhuang Zhou or Zhuangzi (c 369–286 BCE), is taken to be the author of the first seven or 'Inner Chapters' of the book that bears his name, the Zhuangzi, (Cooper, 2018: 49; Graham1989, p. 3). Graham writes of Zhuangzi's freedom, 'his irreverent humour and awe at the mystery and holiness of everything', his 'effortless mastery of words and contempt for the inadequacy of words' and his 'bottomless scepticism' (1989, p. 4). Zhuangzi's writings are 'obscure, fragmented, but pervaded by the sensation, rare in ancient literatures, of a man jotting the living thought at the moment of its inception' (1989, p. 48). To the extent that we are often seized by wonder, find ourselves both preoccupied with and disdainful of words and speaking, sceptical of theories and people who seem to be convinced by them, and more interested in staying with the 'living thought' as they arise, rather than the systems that are said to explain them, we are preceded by Zhuangzi.

Zhuangzi speaks about speaking and the limitations of speaking, abandoning ourself to words and abandoning words sometimes for spirited spontaneous action. Like a person speaking freely, he tells us what one person said to another person about something a third person has said about a saying. He tells us what the third person said about the saying, followed by his response to the saying. Then he says, 'How does it seem to you?' (1989, p. 59). As if living thoughts and saying something might evoke living thoughts and saying something. For him, 'success' is a common word for a common failure, and to seek to stand over and above the world as master and owner betrays a failure to begin to understand how we are part of it, what we owe to it and ourself.

A backdrop and counterpoint to the meetings remembered, repeated and reflected on below and philosophical Daoism as I have just outlined it, is Europe's swooping down on peoples and places, its conquest of the earth and acquisition of empires, which began in the fifteenth century. So when Descartes wrote in 1637 that the still 'new sciences' would help us to reach conclusions in life that are of 'greater usefulness', conclusions we can 'apply' 'and thus make ourselves masters and owners of nature' (Descartes, 1637/1977, p. 46), he was writing at a time when the mastery and ownership of peoples and lands was already a social and political reality. This way of engaging with the world seeks to master, dominate, and exploit it, others and even ourself: digging, drilling, always seeking to transform what we find into something fabulous, as if searching everywhere to find or become *El Dorado*, 'the golden one'.

The conviction that all can and must be measured, mapped and manipulated has a vast history and is in the background as well as the foreground of my experience of psychotherapy with a fourteen year old boy.

Finishing school

Sitting in front of me in his school uniform, clean white shirt and school tie, John epitomised the polite, appropriate, 'well brought up', grown up, serious and businesslike young man in a school suit, who had come to an interview with an expert in order for his problem to be identified, so that it could be swooped down on and taken possession of. I do not try to tell him that I do not have much in the way of claws or an eagle's eyes and forcefulness: I have an attentiveness that floats, settles, then finds itself elsewhere. Sometimes the sequence seems to have a sense.

Without conveying that he has any appetite or interests, he tells me, as if both of us or 'one' should be impressed, that after being asked to leave 'a very good school', Dad got him into 'a good school'. However, he continues, there is some indication that he might be asked to leave there too. I play with possible responses, moving from one to another, settling briefly but not settling for what I settle on. I learned that 'a very good school' means something like, 'a school that is expensive, that has many people competing for each place, that has pupils who live on the premises, that sends many pupils to 'good universities', that has quite a few famous former pupils, as well as people who are not famous but very successful in their 'profession'. This sounded like a finishing school for boys, teaching them how to behave and get ahead in the world. I ask how he makes sense of what happened, and might be happening again.

After claiming not to know, and going silent, he eventually revealed that in both cases he got himself into trouble for 'silly pranks'. Tight lipped and cagey, he eventually mumbled something about a 'prank' where an object (or objects?) was placed on a door in order for it to fall on the head of whoever opened the door. He also mentioned moving a chair just as someone tried to sit on it. Then he seemed to seal his mouth and disappear inside himself.

Waiting, abandoned by him – by his abandonment of words – I fall into my own thoughts and responses, as if into an ocean, and it is not clear whether I am swimming or drowning. Can I remember exactly what occurred to me? No, but here are the sorts of thoughts and memories he stirred up in me: that I usually find 'pranks' cruel rather than funny, that when I was his age, I was a black boy at a school for boys who were referred to as 'doubly disadvantaged', that a boy from 'a very good school', who used terms such as 'crikey', 'chaps' and 'chappesses', introduced me to the word 'jape' as a term for a 'prank' or 'joke', that words and speaking are strange, that we might learn to speak and listen in the way that we are spoken and listened to, that the silence has a particular quality. I also dreamt something up. I saw John about five years older, walking along in the town of one of our 'very best' universities. He was not alone but part of a pack of young men who looked exactly like him. Puzzled by this experience, I am suddenly aware that he is back in the room with me, looking at me, and claiming that he does not know what to say. But then he shows me that he does know, although he may need time to find it for himself.

As I remember it, he tells me that he lives with his father and stepmother, his own mother was a controlling domineering person who became even more tyrannical, needing to master and in this way possess everything and everyone, and although Dad pleaded with her and stayed for years, when John was about five, Dad could not take it anymore and left.

I remarked that his father had not only left his mother: his father left him too. He agreed that if his father left his mother, and he, John, was living with his mother, then, yes, his father left him. Not sure whether he was being logical or patronising or agreeable, I said that I meant that he might have feelings about his father leaving him to cope with his mother; he might have been angry with his dad for going. Looking at me as if he had no idea why I might say something so daft and wrong, he told me many things designed to put me right: Dad wanted to take him but mother would not have this; Dad visited; he could see why Dad left her; he would have, had he been able to, and so on.

When he claimed that of course he missed his father, as he 'liked having him around', I felt that he was managing to 'protest too much' and too little at the same time. He did not actually say, 'Don't be stupid!' but he insisted, Dad was right to go, and no, he was not angry with his father for leaving.

Continuing to build a strong case to prove that he did not have strong feelings about his father's departure, he tells me that when Dad came to visit, he, John, went upstairs to play by himself in his room, and this shows, he claimed, that he was not really bothered by Dad's going or visiting.

As he spoke, I imagined him in his room acting as if he might be playing, but listening out for the music of the exchange between the adults downstairs, and hoping to hear the heavy bass footsteps of an adult male ascending the staircase. Something descended in me as I had this image, something like crushing disappointment.

So, prompted by my imagination, by my wandering off after abandoning myself to him and his words, I said that this left me thinking that no one came upstairs to find out if he was alright or if he was upset. Although he he did not speak, but looked at me as if he had no idea what I was talking about, I felt that he wanted to know how I could know that. I continued by saying that his leaving the sitting room downstairs could be taken as an indication that he was angry or upset. My saying this only resulted in his redoubling his efforts to get me to see that he was relatively indifferent to his father going and arriving. Then he stopped suddenly and said something like, 'I just remembered'. When his father was leaving the house after that visit, John came out of his room upstairs and threw his toy truck downstairs at his father's head. He grinned as he told me this. 'Remembering' here seems to have much to do with seeing how things might be related, with acknowledging the importance of something, rather than just retrieving information: it seemed as if he was conceding that he could see that there was something in the idea that he was angry with his father for going. I asked him if this had the desired effect. What did his father do? Dad raced upstairs and spent a long time shouting at him for his stupid and dangerous behaviour. I said, 'So you got him to come upstairs and stay there shouting at you?' John wanted to say more about this, but I ended the session because it was time. He did not look happy.

This meeting took place in a service that was becoming increasingly subject to measurement, with a battery of evaluation forms being given to 'clients' or rather 'customers'. I imagined being summonsed by a young manager, who after quoting the current guidelines would also recite all of the ways I had fallen short with this client. I did not say much when the client wanted me to get on with it; I probably looked distracted or sleepy sometimes. Then I talked about his father, although he told me that what I said was wrong and seemed to indicate that I was a bit stupid. Then I stopped the session when, more engaged and fluid, he wanted to talk.

At the beginning of his second session, in spite of my attempts to help him to speak, he again looked quite lost and resourceless, and I felt as if I was being cruel for not helping him more, as if I was playing a 'prank' by not speaking more, as if he was the victim of my cruelty. Again he disappeared into himself, returned, then did not know what to say. Then he changed and seemed to have quite a bit to say, accompanied by quite a lot of grinning, and a sense in me that he was more candid and real.

He had been thinking about the previous session: his throwing his truck at his father's head. It was the first time Dad had visited since he left. As he acknowledged and apparently enjoyed that his actions had detained his father, I caught a glimpse of how 'chucking' his truck at his father's head – like a fisherman hooking and reeling in a fish – might be connected to resting objects on doors so they might fall on someone's head. I started to wonder about the sense of his actions and repetition. What was he doing to Dad then and to the other boys now? Heads are hurt or damaged? He protested, though, as if catching himself enjoying the memory was clearly not right. The serious and proper young man was back and claiming that remembering his misbehaviour then does not help him with his problems now. It was not, he said, 'relevant'. In this climate, the 'r' word might have intimidated me, but missing the threat, I said I thought he could not say much when he was a small child about feeling angry, missing his father, feeling as if he is not being listened to, but he knew how to get people to scream and shout at him. The problem seems to be that he is good at this, but not good at trying to tell them why he may be upset and angry. This seemed to me to be part of the problem at his schools and at home. It was not as if what he remembered and repeated to me belonged only to the past; it seemed as if these issues were very much alive and he was repeating them in his actions.

John never missed a session, nor was he ever late. His sessions were littered with what I experienced as his abandoning speaking or being abandoned by the capacity to speak: there were despairing silences, emptiness, disappearances, drifting, sometimes drowning. I found myself being careful and slow, although I knew that we would not have very much time. I feared violating him by talking too much at him, pushing him to answer my questions, respond to my comments, covering over what is there with grown up words. Eventually, I began to wonder about my not wanting to be like the domineering mother who has to control everything, or the father who does not respond to his wordless distress and needs but may shout at him and deliver monologues, and how the 'very good school' and the 'good school' might be experienced as echoes of these experiences.

I sat with his disappearance, berated myself for not helping him more, and therefore being cruel, drifted off myself and imagined him with the same group of lads who looked just like him, out drinking at the 'very good' university. He was laughing, carrying on, performing, but he did not seem to be happy.

Sometimes from these silences he seemed to hook something that had some meaning for him and would speak with interest and feeling. During these times, I felt hopeful; but often I worried about doing too much, dominating, interfering, and about abandoning him, either by speaking and overvaluing speaking, encouraging him to behave like a big boy who can speak and abandon his silence, or abandoning him by not talking to him in a way that made it easier for him to speak back to me. When I broke a long silence early in a session with 'You are very quiet!', he told me that people often say he is, and often he does not know what to say. I expressed curiosity about his apparent disappearances. He said he knew what I meant. He did not understand what happened to him. He did not know what to say. He was worried about these disappearances, worried that there was something wrong with him, but he could not seems to utter more words about this.

Things improved at home and at school. John became more willing and able to talk, rather than meeting others with long silences, grunts, one word responses, and the silly pranks that got him into trouble, especially at school. He was more responsive to invitations to conversations and even initiated some himself.

One session, after his usual silence and wandering off, he began to speak quickly and with feeling about the latest laptop, how great it was, its beautiful lines and how he and his friends (a group of fourteen to fifteen year olds boys) had been reading and talking about it for months, dreaming of getting their hands on it. He told me that the morning the laptop came out, he was 'shocked' to hear his stepmother speak about it with enthusiasm to his father as they were at breakfast. He had, he said, no idea that she had any idea about such things. Then Dad started to ask her about it like he was interested. John said he found it 'surreal' to listen to his stepmother and father talk about things that he did not really think they knew about or were interested in. John sounded as if he thought his generation had invented interest, longing, desiring, and, therefore, sex. 'You'll never guess what happened next!' he exclaimed, in a way that made it clear that I was not really being invited to guess. The next evening, his father turned up with one of these new laptops for his stepmother, who was really excited by and appreciative of what he had given to her. Something about the way he looked at me, expressing surprise, indignation, maybe confusion, prompted me to say, as if for him, 'What about me?' Looking directly at me, showing and expressing that this is unbelievable, and words almost fail him entirely, he utters, 'That's well over a grand! She only has to mention it!'

Giving myself over to what he had to say about his father and stepmother, their giving and receiving, pleasure and excitement with each other, as if I am being told about their abandon with each other, I find myself taking up the issue of his feeling abandoned or left out, and remark that his father had a different relationship with his stepmother, compared to the one he had with his son. I said also that I wonder whether he, John, worried that his stepmother might not want him there sometimes.

Looking surprised, John grinned and said that in a recent argument between them, he had said just this to her, and rather than being very angry with him, as he expected, she seemed to be hurt and assured him that this was his home. I was reassured by what I heard as talk about 'sex', rivalry and engagement rather than withdrawal and cruel 'pranks', yet plagued by the sense that the story about the laptop was a gift to me that I failed to accept well. For clearly this very quiet boy, who often did not know what to say or often abandoned words, had suddenly spoken with abandon, and I wanted him to hear that I had heard him and that his words had not just been abandoned.

Things continued to go well. Still quiet with a tendency to disappear, he had things to say sometimes, and would listen to what I had to say about his silences, his leaving others by disappearing and his 'pranks', which I thought had something to do with his feelings about being left alone, feeling stupid, bad, unhappy, angry, as if something cruel was being done to him, and his difficulties abandoning himself to speaking, rather than acting under the influence of how he felt. He went from silence in the face of my comments to trying to speak about his confusion, puzzlement and concerns about his silences, disappearances and finding himself in trouble.

In a service concerned with efficiency and effectiveness, measuring rather than getting the immeasurability of things, if there are indications that things are not going well, you might be encouraged to follow the evidence and end the therapy. If things go well, you might be encouraged to end the therapy. For, the argument may go, if he is doing so well then he is clearly not that 'disturbed' and in need – there are other people waiting to be seen – and your hanging on to him indicates your commitment to long term work and making people dependent on psychotherapy. In this context, John and I agreed on a date to end. He said he thought therapy was helping. There had not been any incidents for some time; he was getting on better with people at school as well as at home, and generally finding it easier to be with and talk to people. He did not know how long he 'needed' to see me for.

Rather than ending with the term and the imminent public holidays, I suggested that we ended three weeks into the new term. He told me in response to my asking that his father would be abroad somewhere quite remote over the holiday period, and his stepmother needed to go and look after a sick relative. 'And what about you?' I asked. John explained that as he could not go with either of the adults, he would board at school for two weeks. I showed my concern and confusion. We had been talking about how when his father leaves and is absent, he, John, feels that absence, feels abandoned, lonely and angry. All of the things that have been most concerning seem to have taken place at school. Now he tells me that his father will be away and out of contact with him for two weeks, and he, John, will be a boarder at his school, and it will be fine. Why does he think it will be?

John said he had not thought about it like that. He looked worried. I tried to discuss it with him. He could not speak or think about it, but fell back on saying, 'It should be alright!' as if repeating the mantra. I eventually suggested that he raised these concerns with his father. In the next session, he told me that he had raised this with Dad; Dad had said that it should be alright, and he, John, did not know what to say next, so he dropped it.

The first session after the break was different. He gave me a picture of his rattling around in a relatively empty school for well over a week, trying and just about managing to cope with his sense of being abandoned and left out of where he would most like to be. On the tenth day his father managed to locate a phone that had some coverage and phoned John, who was very pleased and excited to hear from him. Immediately after the phone call he did something dangerous to the school, the other people in it and himself. He had to leave the 'good school'.

He could say little about this event initally. I spoke to him about his anger with the school and his father, his holding these feelings in and being disconnected from them, and how they came to the surface after he said goodbye to his father at the end of the call. He listened, did not look bewildered, and joined in, as if piecing together with me me for the first time, something he knew but had not formed words for.

Dressed casually now, as he no longer needed to be in uniform, he seemed more able to speak freely. By the week after, his penultimate session, he had a place at the local school. This meant no uniform, no getting up very early and having to take trains and buses to school, whilst loaded up like a pack-horse. This lighter boy, freer in himself, was more able to acknowledge his angry despairing feelings around the things that happened at home with his mother, his father leaving him, the schools for conquistadors with their rules, regulations, expectations and traditions, set on producing prominent and prosperous people, whilst being oppressive, unable to listen and not seeming to care, rather like his first home. At the end of his final session he surprised me by saying with feeling that he wishes that we did not have to end, that it was a shame.

Conquistador questions and preoccupations, conformity and compliance

If we listen with some abandon to this account of listening with some abandon, and becoming freer to abandon oneself to and in speaking, we might hear ourself wonder about 'conquistador questions and preoccupations', and whether such questions and preoccupations might be heard as repeating rather than remembering and trying to 'work through' – in the sense of steadily illuminating, or keeping in our gaze, or not just staying stuck in repeating (Freud, 1914) – a crucial part of our history. We might wonder whether this repeating is evident in neoliberalism: the position or conviction that human wellbeing is best served by individual entrepreneurial freedom, which emphasises property and property rights, efficiency, competition, measurable outcomes, equating a good life with 'success', 'high performance' and significant financial gain (Kelly & Moloney, 2018, pp. 84–85), with finding or becoming 'the golden one'.

'Conquistador questions' about my meetings with this boy may include questions about the financial cost of the therapy, its cost efficiency and effectiveness, and how we know or prove anything here. We are also asking 'conquistador questions' when we ask who this account belongs to. Does it belong to the service where the work was carried out? Does it belong to John or his legal guardian? Whose property is it? Who is the master and possessor here?

If I am writing about my experience of being with John, or rather my remembering this experience now and what I made of it – or what I make of what I made of it – do we have to answer what I am referring to as 'conquistador questions' by claiming that I am the master and possessor of my own remembering – and therefore perhaps my own forgetting – repeating or retelling? It might be possible to say that these acts of remembering, repeating, the way I experience, certainly are mine, but I do not stand to them in the relationship of master and possessor. Rather they are mine or of me in the way that how I move, how I laugh and at what, my shadow and my footprints are mine.

More interesting to a psychotherapist than questions about measurement, mastery and ownership might be questions about my remembering and repeating here, and what I might be understood as trying to 'work through' in what I have written (S Freud, 1914; Phillips, 2016). Why this boy rather than another? Surely **how** I experience, **what** I remember and, therefore, fail to remember, is of me and crucial?

Before making an attempt to begin to follow such thoughts about what this particular therapist may be remembering, and repeating, working through or failing to work through when he wants to think of himself as hard at work, it may be important that we give a little consideration to **our** 'finishing schools', and not only those attended by our clients.

If there are over 500 types of psychotherapy being practiced today (David et al., 2016, p. 6), there are many 'finishing schools' for psychotherapists, teaching people how to see the world correctly, convinced that they are part of a 'good' or 'very good school' and that someone should be impressed. They are places for conferring on students the right to present and even think of themselves as 'experts', as masters and possessors of a body of knowledge or set of skills. And these places are schools that might 'finish a person off'. Are there many places where it is possible to engage in an education in listening and speaking, rather than a training on what you should hear and how, what you should say and how?

In these schools and in the journals they read and write, there are clearly currently two ways of writing about psychotherapeutic experiences. One way is to set out our theoretical resources before applying them to examples of client work. Another way is to begin with client work before reaching for the theoretical resources to illuminate or explain.

Complying with one of these popular plots and producing something that might claim to be a 'scientific paper' is one option now. However, if this piece of writing claims that there are campaigns against compliance and the overvaluation of technological thinking in Zhuangzi, Nietzsche and some versions of psychoanalysis, alongside an appreciation of the story and the way it is told, as well as odes to appetite and the enjoyment of life, it is perhaps fitting that at this point it does not comply with how things are usually done, that it is wary of making claims about being 'scientific' and 'technological', but is more interested in the tale and the telling of the tale.

Rather than being preoccupied with 'applying' theory, we might be interested in what might contribute to our becoming a person to whom a theory or particular way of looking and being might 'call'. What predisposes us to some theories and perspectives and to find others indigestible or laughable? Why might we look to some sentences as saviour or salvation, as escape from the hermeneutic circle of making sense, or the 'deus ex machina' who appears towards the end of the play, solving the apparently insoluble, fixing the apparently unfixable? If we do not see like gods or eagles, but as human beings at a particular time, in a particular place, and our seeing is related to our horizons, impulses, errors, ideals and fantasies, our needs and desires (F Nietzsche, 1887: sections 120 and 125), we may try to say a little about our seeing, what calls to us and why.

Does it need to be stated that all accounts are selective, partial, subject to memory, desire and the occasion, always leaving something out, and revealing in a particular way? Nothing has been said, for example, about the part played by John's uncle and his being an only child. Little has been said about his 'disappearances'. Some things are explicit, easier to interrogate and measure, but what lurks, threatens and fails to materialise may also be very important.

Here is an attempt to say something about what might lie behind or beneath my listening and speaking to this boy in this way, as well as the ideas and concepts used and appealed to in this paper. In other words, what might we say about this piece of writing in terms of what it remembers and expresses, fails to remember and give expression to?

Fishing

When I was a small boy on one of those Caribbean islands, first claimed by Spain near the beginning of the sixteenth century, then taken by force by Britain towards the end of that century, I would listen to my grandfather's stories about being out on a boat on the ocean, fishing. Freely floating out where there is no sight of land, where the sun is often merciless and the weather may suddenly lose her temper, the creatures in the water grow huge, wild, strong and mean. And you can never know what has taken hold of your line. It might be a swordfish or shark, ferocious, spoiling to fight and bite. (Every child knows that a 'swordfish' has a sword and is only too eager to use it.) It might be a monster from the depth that no human being has ever seen and lived to tell the tale.

Listening to words I could barely understand and imagining what I had never see, I abandoned myself to the oceans of words, images and gestures that flowed from this master of storytelling. The mistake most people make, he told me, slowly and deliberately, as if warning me not to be stupid enough to fall for this too, is that as soon as they feel that something might be on the end of their line, they begin to yank and pull and haul, seeking to overpower what may be there, show it who is boss. But this is precisely what you must not do.

For if you do this and you are lucky, your line, your link with this unknown creature will snap, and you will never know what might have been had you managed not to behave like a brawling idiot. If you are not so lucky, you might be pulled into the water, becoming food for the vicious shark or sea serpent. The person who is wise in this situation has learned to feel and to respond to cues and clues. Such a person might respond to a tug on the line by doing nothing, or even by letting the line out so that whatever is on the end of it feels free to run and jump and fight. There is a right time for tempting all that tugs unseen in the water, to show itself on deck. This is learnt and can be taught by people who who have cultivated this ability. But the person who is able to give a good account of what needs to be done is not necessarily a good teacher of this art. The person who knows all the Latin names for what lives in the oceans and how to classify all creatures is also not necessarily a good teacher of waiting and cunning and something forceful at the right time. Mastery is part of it but being intent on crude control and domination of other living things is not where you should be. What is crucial has more to do with letting go, with the capacity to flow with what is happening, to follow faithfully rather than impose oneself, interfere and try to command.

It is possible to stand on deck, rod in hand, singing a song about ruling the waves and nearly a third of the earth. This is different from thinking of oneself as a reader of signs, of wind and waves and what lurks unseen.

In this allegory, what is in the sea does not necessarily stand in for what is in the unconscious part of the client's psychical apparatus or even my own. If we follow Heidegger rather than Freud, it stands for what has not been laid out clearly on the deck or shore and is being examined in the light of day (Heidegger, 1962). The sea and its content is the background that allows all things to be as they are, that allows us to float, feeling confident that we know where we are and what is what. It includes cultural and political factors, such as notions of 'good schools' and who goes to boarding school. It is where we cannot see, including what we may glimpse but slips and evades our direct examination. It contains too, what may be beyond our capacity to see and know: what seems inexplicable and wondrous.

If this story about a story and its reverberations can be accepted as an allegory rather than a theory or theoretical model, we might not entangle ourself in trying to state exactly how it fits the practice of psychotherapy or how it gives practitioners the power to predict and control, or how exactly it is to be applied to the account above. It does not have to be the case that the client or patient is the fish the practitioner hooks and reel in. It is possible to say that there are hooks and bait for both of them. One of them might be working to bring something to light, on the clearing of the deck, whilst the other is doing their best to keep it in the water. And sometimes, at least, it is a matter of cooperation, of the two working together reeling as they reel in: befuddled, muddled and bemused, bewitched, distracted and off balance as they try to call and recall, to pull in and pull up, to take up and take back whatever seems to be on lines that are repeatedly snapped. But this is a strange kind of fishing, for although the lines have creatures or living experiences on them and are tangled up in other lines, it is not clear where a line ends, what is connected to what, or if there can be much more than reeling together.

These two tales about fishing, imagining, reading signs, and the importance of following and facilitating rather than controlling and possessing, are in contrast to 'conquistador questions and preoccupations', and already reveal much about Daoism, existentialism and psychoanalysis. The first tale is of a boy who begins his sessions 'correct' in the sense of 'proper', and in search of information. It soon seems that pressure to conform, his difficulties expressing himself, his making a foreigner of the anger and destructiveness he is in danger of feeling, are all important and interrelated. In his case, it is possible that his 'finishing school' may be too much for him, may 'finish him off'. There is some reading, waiting and slowly drawing closer to what seems to be lurking. There is some getting tangled up in the session, a little force in a particular direction, and quite a lot of trying to follow the cues and clues. 'Cure' is not obviously a good word for what takes place. There is a little more freedom, more talking, or things just 'coming up': there is more of a sense that the bringing things up together is more to the point than his being given information, and that this is a way of coming to deciding and acting.

Flourishing

Zhuangzi, Nietzsche, Heidegger and some versions of psychoanalysis are explicitly and consistently against intellectualising and over theorising our experience, and against compliance. Life is to do with engagement, pleasure, wonder, yet 'society' or 'culture' wrestles from us our pleasures, interests and sense of wonder in order to give us pleasures, interests and aims that are more advantageous to it (Freud, 1908, 1930). This emphasis on our lived experience of being engaged in the world and our capacity to do so whole-heartedly, creatively and skilfully – rather than our cleverness, capacity for calculation, our ability to be rational according to the standards of others around us – is something found in Daoism, existentialism and some versions of psychoanalysis (Nietzsche 1887: section 125; Spelman 2013: 177).

David Cooper states

'The sense of "harmony with the cosmos" and the depreciation of theoretical knowledge, then, are not two distinct ingredients ... For the reverse side of that depreciation is the elevation of another mode of knowledge which is a style of harmonious engagement with the world.' (Cooper, 2003, p. 65).

These critiques of knowingness, of overvaluing knowing, of our craving for calculative knowledge, are warnings about and an appreciation of limits, our limits and the poverty of gathering mountains of facts, true statements, knowledge (Cooper, 2018, p. 50), just the sort of information needed by would be masters and possessors. Heidegger states, 'the will to make and be effective, has overrun and crushed thought' (Heidegger, 1968, p. 25). Psychoanalysis is at least a claim that we are impoverished and impoverishing if we cling only to what is rational, conscious, clear and well thought out. It is at least a claim that as well as dealing with texts there are subtexts, pretexts, talk is textured; as well as light there is darkness, shade and shadow. It is at least a way of warning us about our tendency to huddle together in the light because we are afraid of what we might have banished and darkened, our tendency to distance ourself from ourself.

Nietzsche tried to tell us in the nineteenth century that science is a way of re-describing the world to help us to exploit it according to the needs and desires we find ourselves with (Nietzsche, 1885/1982; section 14). Seducing and distracting us with promises of what we can have and do, science succeeds too well in helping to spread forgetfulness and inattentiveness over the gods we worship, the lives we actually live, the experiences we have, the values and goals we cling to – often with little serious thought – as they are often repeatedly supported and reinforced around us (Cooper 1983). Nietzsche as well as Husserl (Loewenthal & Snell, 2003) urges us to learn to bracket or put out of play what we take ourselves to know, to be so well educated that we are able to think little of our education (Nietzsche, 2004). What we take ourselves to know is often not what we have experienced, not what we have been deeply shaken by, but what we have been taught, how we have been educated, what we conform to. Here is the idea that our schooling might finish us off by enforcing compliance without appetite, interest or thought.

Zhuangzi seems to say that this preoccupation with knowing, learning and measuring prepares and enables us to exercise and be swallowed up by our greed (Zhuangzi chapter 10). He produces a sustained opposition to imposing human goals on nature and our dependence on and infatuation with the technology which springs form this calculative knowledge. It is this form of knowledge that enables us to 'interfere' in a rough, witless and oafish way with all the world (Cooper , 2018:51; Z 13;). He claims that we interfere with and mistreat ourselves. The Zhuangzi states,

The energy of life is limited. The mind is insatiable. To put a limited instrument at the discretion of an insatiable master is always risky, and often fatal. The master will wear out the instrument . Prolonged, exaggerated intellectual effort uses up life (Zhuangzi chapter 3).

Zhuangzi is clear that we human beings court disaster by insisting on interfering in everything, violating whilst being convinced that we are doing good, bringing order to chaos, making things as we think they should be, making them 'perfect' and 'artificial', so they cease to be what they were (Zhuangzi chapter7).

Daoism contains a reminder of how we are easily seduced by language (Zhuangzi chapter 2), which is an important theme in Nietzsche (Nietzsche, 1873, for example), as well as in Wittgenstein, Heidegger, and explicitly in some versions of psychoanalysis (Phillips, 1998, for example), in so far as words are what the others, 'they', the adults use and we or 'the child' must fall in with the order of the words around and in us.

In the Zhuangzi, there is a consistent critique of conformity as what helps us to close our eyes to ourselves (Zhuangzi chapter 31). A similar critique of conformity along with enticement and encouragement towards taking one's existence seriously can be found throughout Nietzsche's writings (for example, Nietzsche, 1874, 1885/1982). Winnicott and Adam Phillips are two psychoanalysts who are preoccupied with 'conformity' or 'compliance'. The movement made by these philosophers and psychoanalysts is away from what demands conformity and compliance and towards some notion of an authentic naturalness and spontaneity that has much to do with being free to wander, roam, not being caught up in limited perspectives.

I have begun to read Zhuangzi as offering us a mocking critique of one version of what it means to be a grown up, of the desire to be master and possessor of nature and the owner of people and parts of the earth. It is ridiculous, he might say, to stand on deck, rod in hand, singing a song about ruling the waves, what we have and our other achievements, but oblivious to coming storms, what lurks unseen, eyes closed to ourself, our shadow and footprints. Daoism seems to say that this desire to know all, have all and be the master is a bad version of what it means to be childish. The child has to learn that it floats on and in something vast and beyond its imagination, and that there are many distractions to take it away from itself.

As well as reading Daoism as a critique of a serious and dominant conception of what it means to be a grown up, it might also be read in terms of parenting and psychotherapy. Daoism is a preoccupation with and hymn to following and receptivity, to enabling, nourishing, facilitating: that is, an engagement with the world and with ourself which is scrupulously concerned with not violating, not trampling on what may be there, being worried about trying to alter or perfect, and the desire to get people and things under our power. *Wu wei*, then, or 'non-action' or 'spontaneity' is to do with following and not violating, 'letting be'. It is a way of respect and reverence to all.

In the first edition of The Gay Science, Nietzsche, quoting Emerson, writes, 'To the poet and the sage, all things are friendly and hallowed, all experience profitable, all days holy, all men divine' (Nietzsche, 1874, p. 8). This may be read as sounding something similar to Daoism, a spirit of reverence and welcome.

Brooks (2008) argues that Nietzsche is close to the ancient sceptics – in his consistent hostility towards theoretical stances, doctrines and dogma – rather than the Cartesian sceptic, who is concerned with certainty and the infallible system. Nietzsche writes,

One should not let oneself be misled: great intellects are sceptics. Zarathustra is a sceptic. The vigour of a mind, its freedom through strength and superior strength, is *proved* by scepticism. Men of conviction simply do not come into consideration where the fundamentals of value and disvalue are concerned. Convictions are prisons ... Freedom from conviction of any kind, the capacity for an unconstrained view, pertains to strength. (Nietzsche, 1888, A, p. 54).

For Nietzsche, philosophy is education towards liberation as freedom from being constrained by the opinions and limited perspectives of others, an inoculation against what is current and dominant (Cooper 1983). From this perspective, dogma and doctrines, convictions, theories and their application can not be what is important in Nietzsche's writings or in psychotherapy. He is concerned with how scrupulous we are about our thinking and our taste and with how we might 'cultivate a capacity for an unconstrained view'. His comments about the poet and the sage above might be considered with or linked to the notion of 'cultivating the capacity for an unconstrained view', if we think that poets and sages cultivate and display this capacity to follow and not violate, to dream with but not be asleep to. Perhaps it is possible to see similarities to what the Daoist sage tries to do through his 'spiritual exercises' that are to help him to wander and roam and not get stuck in the perspectives he finds around and within him (Cooper, 2018, p. 51). Is it possible to regard free association as Freud conceived it (Freud, 1912) as a 'spiritual exercise', as a setting sail together, wary of 'lazy peace, from cowardly compromise' (Nietzsche, 1888) and the constrains we are tempted to comply with?

If the Zhuangzi shows us 'happy meandering . . . in the midst of life' and its problems (Wu, 1982, p. 14) and aims to 'evoke the reader into coming to grips with himself', to 'self-scrutiny' (Wu, 1982, p. 8), its affinities with existentialism and psychoanalysis might be easily seen.

To meander, float or wander is different from running away. In some versions of therapy and philosophy, we often seek to transform being in flight from or oblivious to, into being able to wander, meander, not know where we are going, to forget ourselves and allow ourself to remember.

For many in the world of psychotherapy, 'the shadow' is a term used by Carl Jung (Jung & Jaffé, 1965). Before Jung, Nietzsche called the second part of Human, All Too Human, 'The Wanderer and His Shadow' (F Nietzsche, 1986). This idea is also in Zhuangzi, for example, in a chapter where Confucius, as if stating his 'presenting problem', what he has come for help with, asks why he repeats the pattern of being 'honoured everywhere, and then persecuted and expelled'. The old fisherman tells him that his problem is that he closes his eyes to himself and opens them too much to others. He then tells Confucius a tale, a parable of a man who was so afraid of his shadow and footprints that he tried to run away from them, to get away and save himself from them, but no matter how fast and single-mindedly he ran, he could not get away from them. And so he died running from his footprints and his shadow.

There may be many objections to what is written here; only two will be touched on briefly. Fishing, it might be objected, is a good example of a conquistador activity. For anglers compete with each other about who can catch the biggest or the most fish. We can fish with dynamite or huge nets, ravaging, depleting and destroying what is around us. The theme of fish, fishing and fishermen in the Zhuangzi, however, seems to have much to do with pleasure and being engaged with the world, others and ourself in a way that is not clean and dead, but alive, muddy and in the moment (Zhuangzi chapter 17). The fisherman is an emblem: one who is able to engage and respond according to the situation, rather than impose himself and dominate. This is to follow the Dao. In the Zhuangzi, the fisherman is not one who amasses more fish than anyone else, more than he can eat, and leaves others to go hungry. The story about a story and its telling remembered above is about learning to wait, listen, abandon oneself to the call of the moment, as well as a passion for listening and speaking.

This paper is written as the coronavirus brings death and anxiety to the world, rudely confronting us with our mortality, vulnerability and limitations. Furthermore, the issue of racism has been highlighted yet again by the murder of a black man at the hands of a group of policemen. Why write about psychotherapy and philosophy at a time like this? Surely they are both irrelevant?

Here are two brief responses. It could be argued that Zhuangzi, Nietzsche and existentialism generally, and psychoanalysis, provide us with relentless reminders that whilst we may not understand well enough what it means to practice 'self-isolation' and 'social distancing', we are experienced wearers of masks and seasoned practitioners of 'self-distancing'. The client work presented, the discussion above, this tale told by an old fisherman and much of psychotherapy might be said to have much to do with our attempt to respond to a tendency to 'self-distancing', to run away from our shadow and footprints, to stand on deck singing a song about what we rule and have, unaware of pandemics and other possible storms.

It may be evident to some readers that power, privilege and race are clearly in this piece of writing, although they have not been dragged on deck to be examined in the light of day. It is possible to be a little more explicit, whilst fearing that the leviathan of racism cannot be hauled onto a small boat without sinking it. I take 'racism' to refer to the actions, beliefs and practices that reflect or support the ideology that human beings can be neatly and scientifically divided into groups, and that there is a causal link between a person's race, on the one hand, and their disposition, intelligence, actions and worth, on the other. It is a way of assuming or claiming, crudely or subtly, whether through mendacity, greed, laziness or ignorance of history, that the possession of resources, wealth and privileges reflects differences between peoples which are scientific, maybe biological, evolutionary or developmental. It is, I am suggesting, a way of repeating and being dominated by our history rather than remembering or reflecting on it. Dalal writes that 'Racism is a form of organising peoples, commodities and the relationship between them by making reference to a notion of race' (2002: 27). Who could think that racism has nothing to do with the shadows and footprints of those who have sought, with a great deal of success, to be masters and possessors of the world, with conquistador convictions and the repeating of this in neoliberalism, that the earth, other people, and even we ourselves are standing resources to be exploited in the name of efficiency, profit and success?

Disclosure statement

No potential conflict of interest was reported by the author.

References

Brooks, O. (2008). "Cultivating the capacity for an unconstrained view": Nietzsche, education and psychotherapy. *Philosophical Practice: Journal of the American Philosophical Practitioners Association*, 3(2), 285–297.

D E, C. (1983). *Authenticity and Learning: Nietzsche'sEducational Philosophy*. Routledge and Kegan Paul.

D E, C. (2003). *World Philosophies: An Historical Introduction* (Second ed.). Blackwell Publishing.

D E, C. (2014). *Daoism, Nature and Humanity', in Anthony O'Hear edited Philosophical Traditions*. Cambridge University press.

D E, C. (2018). *Zhuangzi and the Meaning of Life', in S Leach and J Tartaglia edited The Meaning of Life and the Great Philosophers*. Routledge.

Dalal, F. (2002). *Race, Colour and the Process of Racialization*. Brunner-Routledge.

David, D., Lynn,, & Montgomery, G. H. (2016). *Evidence-Based Psychotherapy: The State of the Science and Practice*. John Wiley and Sons inc.

Descartes, R. (1637/1977). Discourse on the method of rightly directing one's Reason and of seeing Truth in the Sciences. In E. Anscombe and P. Geach (Eds.), *Philosophical writings* (pp. 5–57). Thomas Nelson and Sons.

Freud, S. 1908. *"Civilized" Sexual Morality and Modern Nervous Illness'. The Standard Edition of the Complete Psychological Works of Sigmund Freud*. Vol. ume IX. 1906-1908. Jensen's 'Gradiva' and Other Works 177–204. London: The Hogarth Press.

Freud, S. 1912. *Recommendations to Physicians Practising Psycho-Analysis'. The Standard Edition of the Complete Psychological Works of Sigmund Freud*. Vol. ume XII. 1911-1913. The Case of Schreber, Papers on Technique and Other Works 109–120. London: The Hogarth Press.

Freud, S. (1914). *Remembering, Repeating and Working Through' (Further Recommendations on the Technique of Psycho-analysis ll). Standard Edition of the Complete Works of Sigmund Freud* (Vol. Xll). London: The Hogarth Press.

Freud, S. (1930). *Civilization and its Discontents*. Penguin Books.

Froese, K. (2006). *Nietzsche, Heidegger and Daoist Thought. Crossing Paths in-Between*. State University of New York Press.

Graham, A. C. (1989). Chuang-Tzu: The Inner Chapters. Unwin Paperbacks

Heidegger, M. (1962). *Being and Time*. Oxford, Blackwell.

Heidegger, M. (1968). *What is Called Thinking?* Harper and Row.

Jung, C. G., & Jaffé, A. (1965). *Memories, Dreams, Reflections*. Random House.

Kelly, P., & Moloney, P. (2018). CBT is the method: The object is to change the heart and soul. In D. Loewenthal & G. Proctor (Eds.), *Why not CBT: Against and For CBT Revisited* (pp. 82–105). PCCS Books.

Loewenthal, D., & Snell, R. (2003). *Post-modernism for psychotherapists*. Brunner-Routledge.

Nietzsche, F. (1873). *On truth and lie in an extra-moral sense', in Walter Kaufman edited The Portable Nietzsche*. Penguin Books.

Nietzsche, F. (1874). *'Schopenhauer as educator' in R J Hollingdale translated, Untimely Meditations*. Cambridge University Press.

Nietzsche, F. (1887). *The Gay Science*. Vintage Books.

Nietzsche, F. (1888). *The Anit-Christ, in R J Hollindale translated Twilight of the Idols and The Anti-Christ*. Penguin Books.

Nietzsche, F. (1982/1885). *Beyond Good and Evil*. Penguin Books.

Nietzsche, F. (1986). *Human, All Too Human: A Book For Free Spirits*. Cambridge University Press.

Nietzsche, F. (2004). *On the Future of our Educational Institutions*. St Augustine's Press.

Parkes, G. (1996). *Nietzsche and Asian Thought*. University of Chicago Press.

Phillips, A. (1998). *The Beast in the Nursery*. Faber and Faber Limited.

Phillips, A. (2016). "On "remembering, repeating and working through, " Again'." *Contemporary Psychoanalysis, 52*(3), 375–382. https://doi.org/10.1080/00107530. 2016.1174812

Spelman, M. B. (2013). *The Evolution of Winnicott's Thinking: Examining the Growth of Psychoanalytic Though Over Three Generations*. London: Karnac Books.

Wu, K. M. (1982). *Chuang Tzu; World Philosopher at Play*. The Crossroad Publishing Company.

Zhuangzi. (1984). *Zhuang Zi in Derek Bryce translation of Leon Wieger's Wisdom of The Daoist Masters*. Llanerch Enterprises.

The golden cage

Bice Benvenuto

ABSTRACT

The key issue of the papers I reviewed seems to lie in the interconnection between therapeutic and social ethos. In fact today malaise is tied to a particular mind-set of our contemporary culture where a distortion of the relations to objects is paramount. This is the double-edged sword of a failure in the construction of the object, which goes hand-in-hand with a failure of a family narrative. The objects of immediate satisfaction such as high tech gadgets and their solitary enjoyment remind me of the autistic spectrum, which has become today mental paradigm, following the decline of past psychic configurations such as classical neurosis or psychosis. Commodity-based and calculative modes of *non-thinking* have become the norm. Symbiotic primary relations do not allow addressing a call towards the other to whom the young is just sticking. The call, stifled by the immediate consummation of commodities, cannot be heard and we are not allowed the time and space to construct our own subjectivity, a space of separation which implies *towardness*.

Der goldene Käfig

ABSTRAKT

Das Hauptthema der von mir besprochenen Arbeiten scheint in der Verbindung zwischen therapeutischem und sozialem Ethos zu liegen. Tatsächlich ist Unwohlsein heute an eine bestimmte Denkweise unserer zeitgenössischen Kultur gebunden, in der eine Verzerrung der Beziehungen zu Objekten von größter Bedeutung ist. Dies ist das zweischneidige Schwert eines Versagens bei der Konstruktion des Objekts, das mit einem Versagen einer Familienerzählung einhergeht. Die Objekte der unmittelbaren Befriedigung wie High-Tech-Geräte und ihr einsamer Genuss erinnern mich an das autistische Spektrum, das heute nach dem Niedergang vergangener psychischer Konfigurationen wie klassischer Neurose oder Psychose zum mentalen Paradigma geworden ist. Rohstoffbasierte und berechnende Modi des Nichtdenkens sind zur Norm geworden. Symbiotische primäre Beziehungen erlauben es nicht, einen Anruf an den anderen zu richten, an dem die Jungen nur festhalten. Der Ruf, der durch die unmittelbare Vollendung von Waren erstickt wird, ist nicht zu hören, und wir dürfen nicht die Zeit und den Raum, um unsere eigene Subjektivität zu konstruieren, einen Raum der Trennung, *in Richtung* impliziert.

La jaula dorada

RESUMEN

El tema clave de los artículos que fueron revisados parece residir en la interconexión entre la ética terapéutica y social. De hecho, hoy en día el malestar está ligado a una mentalidad particular de nuestra cultura contemporánea donde una distorsión de las relaciones con los objetos es primordial. Esta es la espada de doble filo de un fracaso en la construcción del objeto, que va de la mano con un fracaso de una historia familiar. Los objetos de satisfacción inmediata como los aparatos de alta tecnología y su disfrute solitario me recuerdan al espectro autista, que se ha convertido hoy en paradigma mental, tras el declive de configuraciones psíquicas pasadas como la neurosis clásica o la psicosis. Los modos de no pensar basados en productos básicos y calculativos se han convertido en la norma. Las relaciones primarias simbióticas no permiten dirigir una llamada hacia el otro a quien los jóvenes simplemente se apegan. La llamada, sofocada por la consumación inmediata de los productos básicos, no puede ser escuchado y no se nos da el tiempo y el espacio para construir nuestra propia subjetividad, un espacio de separación que implica *ir hacia*.

La gabbia d'oro

La questione chiave degli articoli che ho esaminato sembra risiedere nell'interconnessione tra ethos terapeutico e sociale. In effetti oggi il malessere è legato a una particolare modalita' mentale della nostra cultura contemporanea in cui gioca un ruolo fondamentale una distorsione delle relazioni con gli oggetti. Questa è la spada a doppio taglio di un fallimento nella costruzione delle relazioni con l'oggetto, che va di pari passo con un fallimento della narrazione familiare. Gli oggetti di immediata soddisfazione come i gadget high-tech e il loro godimento solitario mi ricordano lo spettro autistico, che è diventato oggi paradigma mentale, a seguito del declino delle configurazioni psichiche del passato come la nevrosi classica o la psicosi. Le modalita' calcolative e consumiste di *non-pensiero* sono diventate la norma. Le relazioni primarie simbiotiche non consentono un appello rivolto all'altro al quale il giovane e' rimasto incollato. Soffocato dall'immediata consumazione di prodotti, l'appello non riesce ad essere ascoltato, e cosi' non ci e' permesso il tempo e lo spazio per costruire la nostra soggettività, uno spazio di separazione che implica un *'andare verso'*.

La cage dorée

La question principale soulevée par les articles composant cette édition spéciale est celle de l'interconnexion entre l'esprit qui sous-tend la thérapie et celui qui sous-tend le social. En fait le malaise actuel est lié à un état d'esprit particulier de notre culture contemporaine où une distorsion de nos relations avec les objets est capitale. C'est l'épée à double tranchant d'un échec dans la construction de l'objet qui va de pair avec un échec du récit familial. Les objets de satisfaction immédiate tels que les gadgets technologiques et leur plaisir solitaire me rappellent le spectre autistique devenu le paradigme mental après le déclin des configurations psychiques du passé comme les classiques névroses et psychoses. Les modes de *non-pensée* basées sur la marchandisation et le calcul sont devenus la norme. Les relations primaires symbiotiques ne permettent pas de s'adresser à l'autre auquel le jeune s'accroche juste. L'appel, étouffé par la consommation immédiate de marchandises, ne peut pas être entendu et il ne nous est pas permis de prendre le temps et l'espace pour construire notre propre subjectivité, un espace de séparation impliquant *un se diriger vers*.

Το χρυσό κλουβί

ΠΕΡΊΛΗΨΗ
Το βασικό θέμα των άρθρων που εξέτασα φαίνεται να είναι η διασύνδεση μεταξύ του θεραπευτικού και του κοινωνικού ήθους. Στην πραγματικότητα η τρέχουσα ανησυχία συνδέεται με μια συγκεκριμένη νοοτροπία του σύγχρονου πολιτισμού, όπου η διαστρέβλωση των σχέσεων με τα αντικείμενα είναι ύψιστης σημασίας. Αυτό είναι το δίκοπο μαχαίρι της αποτυχίας στην κατασκευή ενός αντικειμένου, η οποία συμβαδίζει με την αποτυχία στην αφήγηση μια οικογένειας. Τα αντικείμενα άμεσης ικανοποίησης, όπως επινοήματα υψηλής τεχνολογίας και η μοναχική τους απόλαυση, μου θυμίζουν το φάσμα του αυτισμού, το οποίο είναι σήμερα νοητικό πρότυπο, ακολουθώντας την εξασθένιση των προηγούμενων ψυχικών διαμορφώσεων, όπως η τυπική νεύρωση ή η ψύχωση. Η εμπορευματοποιημένη και υπολογιστική στάση του μη-σκέφτεσαι έχουν γίνει ο κανόνας. Οι συμβιωτικές πρωταρχικές σχέσεις δεν επιτρέπουν το κάλεσμα στον άλλον, στις οποίες οι νέοι απλά προσκολλούνται. Το κάλεσμα, που πνίγεται από της άμεσης ικανοποίηση μέσω των εμπορευμάτων, δεν μπορεί να ακουστεί και δεν μας επιτρέπεται ο χρόνος και ο χώρος να κατασκευάσουμε την δική μας υποκειμενικότητα, ένας χώρος διαχωρισμού που υπονοεί *πηγαίνοντας προς*.

SCHLÜSSELWÖRTER Sofortige Befridiegung; Beweisbasiert; Autismus Spektrum; *der Annäherung*; einen Anruf antworten

PALABRAS CLAVE Satisfacción inmediata; basato en evidencias; espectro autista; ir hacia; atender una llamada

PAROLE CHIAVE Soddisfazione immediata; basata sull'evidenza; spettro dell'autismo; andare verso; rivolgere un appello

MOTS-CLÉS satisfaction immédiate; basée sur la preuve; spectre autistique; se diriger vers; adresser un appel

ΛΈΞΕΙΣ ΚΛΕΙΔΙΆ Άμεση ικανοποίηση; ερευνητικά τεκμηριωμένο; φάσμα αυτισμού; *πηγαίνοντας προς*; διαχείριση καλέσματος

At first I found it striking that the subject of this conference regarding work with young adults seemed to summon the necessity of a therapeutic ethos. This made me wonder why the call for an ethos was so fundamental in work with the young compared to adults or children. As we have seen in the papers here collected, ethos takes on a special relevance in relation to Social Ethos. It seems that when working with the young we feel a moral responsibility towards a mind still in construction, at the mercy of both the virtues and the vices of a social context, which can offer guidance and wellbeing as well as corruption.

The stakes of the conference's endeavour are laid down very clearly in Dal Loewenthal's editorial. What is at stake is the ethos of our contemporary culture, of society at large. "Modern technological society is responsible for generating very particular kinds of distress in danger to become normalised." Therefore the values and demands of a society based on commodification and commercialization are paramount not only with regard to the malaise it causes the young but also to a formatting of the very mind of a society, a normalization of its toxicity. So it seems that we are faced with a double-edged danger: "the brain not being able to adjust to being exposed to market forces and pressures from social media" as Loewenthal points out, and the mind of young adulthood becoming too well adjusted to such pressures. A technological global conformism makes us enjoy a wealth of objects we adjust to more or less passively. *The integrated hedonism of homo felix* as the psychoanalyst Massimo Recalcati defines it, but a hedonism which takes a toll. It generates a distress that leads to symptoms that are typical of our era and which I like to call 'contemporary symptoms', insofar as they do not fit classical clinical structures such as neurosis or psychosis. Loewenthal mentions some of these: substance use, violence, self-harm, depression. However I would like to bring to the forth one I tend to consider the paradigm of both our era's pathology as well as the underlying setup of our contemporary mind: autism, which throughout its large spectrum unfurls from the most concerning autism of children to the no less frequent autism among adults and young people. The latter is less detectable, as adults have grown to adjust to the demands of the external world on their eccentric solipsism.

Before unravelling the significance of autism I would like to respond first to the second theme of the conference, concerning the issues involved when working therapeutically with the young. If we take the social dimension as determinant in forming the mindset of the young (and not only them!) I very emphatically agree with Loewenthal's suggestion of a therapeutic psychosocial approach to the young's distress. I have myself applied a social approach to my own work with children by setting up what is known as Maison Verte (Hall et al., 2009; Owen et al., 2017), a place inspired by French psychoanalyst Françoise Dolto, who created a space on the street where any adult accompanied by a child could drop in and be free to stay and play, interact or do nothing with their own and/or other children and adults. It was conceived as a public place, like an *agora*, the ancient Greek public square. Even though it was announced as preventative work against the distress of both children and their young parents, the experience demonstrated that prevention is already an all-round therapy for everyone involved, including the MV hosts! Far from the one-to-one private dialogue of bourgeois settings of traditional psychotherapy, the work relied on the *polylogue*, the Babel of tongues. It relied on babies' early lallations as well as the unfolding of primary relations through pleasures in playing, acting, speaking and listening amongst all ages and all walks of life. And if you are a psychoanalyst you witness and learn how *the opening of the unconscious* arises with the pleasure of being with others. This experience may come close to Loewenthal's idea that the therapeutic ethos of educational and social experiences should be addressed to our wider culture, the idea that public activities and services can make a move towards new ethical choices vis-à-vis the troubled minds of the young. Unfortunately this was not the fate of the Maison Verte-UK, which stopped receiving funds when standardized criteria for funding children services became the norm. The norm requested 'evidence-based' results, forms filled with numbers, statistics and personal information, packaged, standardized and easy to unwrap commodities; and no matter how much I tried to negotiate and show them the worldwide literature on Dolto's project, it was to no avail. As the Maison Verte considered the funders' demands a corrupting of the therapeutic ethos we decided to terminate the project.

I gather from the papers I read also a similar strong criticism of the proceedings of an object-orientated society in its 'consumerising of human experience', as Rowan Williams defines it. His text addresses more specifically the question of time, the necessity of its sequence in the process of psychic growth as opposed to the evacuation of time when the consummation of the commodity must occur in no time. He continues: "We like the sense of immediacy that we are offered by this stress on good experience, the sense of cutting out the interfering middle layers to secure access to what we want."

There is always a gap, however small, between our wish and the satisfaction afforded by the wished-for object. It is in this waiting time that we have to invent strategies to tolerate frustration. Even babies may seem to cry as if demanding immediate gratification from their mother's objects of satisfaction: the breast, a clean nappy etc., rather than call for her reassuring wished-for warm presence. Babies are very good at creating phantasy or transitional objects or even at hallucinating them to meet their wishes, not for the object in itself, but for representing the mother's emotional/sensory connection. Most psychoanalytical orientations seem to agree that the object is not simply the object of need but is representative of a mother who makes those objects meaningful and satisfying. In other words the m/other is not just the carrier of the needed object but the person we *go towards*, who gives a temporal and spatial order and meaning to our primordial objects, a human order where objects have both a personal and shared value.

This is quite different from the objects as 'enjoyed' in the autistic mode, where even people are part of a series of objects ready for use, guarantors of an identical repetition of that use. Nothing has to change because their existence depends on the sameness of naked objects. There is no call towards others, there is no state of *towardness*, either a stopgap or absolute absence, no mental elaboration traverses the middle layers. I take this description as the template of the state of our mind today, whether in a pathological way or, even worse, a normalized one: the young who spend most of their time in their room in front of a gadget screen, possibly on the dole and typically with one parent behind the scenes that feeds and is fed by their mere presence, a mere possession that never changes or moves. As Williams stresses, there is lack of narrative, which can unfold through the time of our unique story or family history, of how we constructed our world, our erotic ties. Williams takes the question from the angle that being human is not 'self-made' but 'being made'. We are made by way of the nature of the primordial bond with a mother and the family story as part of a larger social story telling.

No surprise if Williams has concerns about the lack of a sense of the future, not only in the young generations but also in those who govern the world, the old! Of course, the old are only a little older, as they already belong to the generations of the decline of history's narrative. We lose the sense of the future because we have wiped out our ties with the past so that we cannot draw the logic of the sequel of time. It is as if the world had begun with mass production and the technological revolution of the last century. They are unquestioned givens, even if the toll it takes is the earth itself.

But luckily memory, even when evacuated, can still return. This seems to be happening now with the history of racism thanks to the toppling down of several statues from their pedestals. The 'Black Lives Matter' movement, unlike the black movements of the past, demands a reconnecting of the present to the past, of today's vexations to their roots in barbarian western slavery. It is not 'ambulance services' that many young people all around the world are demanding now, but a lifting of historical repression, the turning over of denial and false conscience. Getting rid of the object-statue, that is, of false idols, may change some of history's fake narratives.

Time is also an important issue in Susan Kegerreis's paper. The point she makes, that child and adolescent psychotherapy training is necessary when working with young adults, for whom "it has not yet been possible to master the challenge of the earlier stage", finds me in total agreement. I would go even further and say that child psychotherapy training should represent a consistent part of any psychotherapy and counselling training, as the mental suffering of adults is mostly a regressive reminder of earlier 'undigested' experiences, just like the vomiting of bulimics!

We have seen in William's paper the double-edged sword of a failure in the construction of the object, which goes hand-in-hand with a failure of a family narrative. Let's see how, following Kegerreis' thoughts.

She is concerned with the sense of time, which pertains especially to adolescents for whom "action can feel less frightening than self-reflection", which is prolonged in older age. The compulsion to act, even by violence or self-harm or even suicide, also beyond adolescence, testifies to a difficulty in overcoming the relational problems arising from the adolescent's difficulty or even impossibility to become an adult, even when they believe they would like to leave that golden cage home can be for them. These strongly emerging symptoms, such as OCD or panic attacks, anorexia and addictions, are characterized by a phobia of moving out or of letting the outside enter their enclosed space, phobia of the *agora* and preservation of the cloister of our solipsism. Some other detains the keys of the cloister/cage, but they are evanescent, do not respond to the child's call because they know what is good for the child: being there to complete their own body and mind. No dialogue needs to develop either with the world or with oneself. Washing hands, shielding with gadgets and screens away from people who are felt like infectious viruses, panic attacks when a job interview or a date is coming up, refusing food or vomiting it, are all acts of refusal, of going on strike, manoeuvres aimed at not encountering an infectious sticky otherness. I would dare saying that acting out or refusing to act – or learn, speak, work, etc. – is antagonistic to the very emerging of an unconscious; the relational conflict is suppressed rather than worked over. These new forms of acting have little to do with the classical Freudian long-winded neurotics.

Still, Kegerreiss highlights the turmoil of the volatile relationship young people have with their super-ego and ego-ideal. Let's try to see in what way this turmoil is different from the Freudian child of last century, who was in antagonism with a father who represented first of all the prohibition of incest, the imago of a ferocious primal figure, a super-ego who could devour his children to prevent being dethroned by them: the god Cronus! But the father (or anyone functioning as a third party) also represents an ideal model, as Kegerreiss points out, to look up to and by whom to be guided in order to gradually move away from a possible mother/child loop-knot. We need help in working over the safe distance to no longer be the mother's main object of enjoyment or the mother being ours.

Even while writing about it, I could see how this family narrative now seems quite far from the reality of our current family structure, one in which the father no longer knows, nor does anyone else, where his place is as regards his children and their mother, who often is not even his partner, as we saw in some clinical snippets from the papers. But even when there is no divorce or separation we witness a decline of the paternal function tout-court. What we call a 'good father' today is usually a motherly one, a replica or a substitute for a somehow wanting mother. I don't mean to say that the mother is symbiotic by definition. On the contrary, many studies from neuroscience and psychoanalysis are now showing that a complex foundational sensory relation to the mother from before birth onwards is crucial to processing otherness and interconnection with the other, and not symbiosis, which is instead a state of failure in the development of primary relations. It is such a failure that has become a main feature of the mindset of our epoch, a feature Kegerreiss sees as linked to an unattainable ego-ideal. I would rather see the ego-ideal as vacant or evanescent, not embodied by a different meaningful third 'presence' that helps to orientate our emotional paths and their ethical configurations.

The children of the new millennium, stuck in their high-tech rooms, panicking and marking their body with self-inflicted wounds, in order to feel they own one, belong psychically to one parent while a consistent third referent, a possible ego-ideal, is vanishing, if not absent. Their role is then reduced to being sucked into a claustrophobic partnership with one parent (sometimes both) to dominate or be dominated by as objects of possession and abuse.

In one of Kegerreiss' cases, the adolescent Marta, while "morphing into an instant adult ... leaping into her sexual life without a care", is acting out indiscriminate sexuality, one that fails to align with the life erotic drive, it cannot reach out towards a desired 'other', but catches on the other's sexed body or high tech gadgets that society feeds to them. They are kept quiet, securely caged to feed their parents' void, so similar to their children's, I'm afraid. In this way the emerging of the subject is compromised, the death drive has gained the upper hand!

My question at this point is: would an excess of object-world entail a shortcoming of subjectivity? Maybe this question is always somehow posed as a criticism by older generations in conflict with the younger ones, at least since the biblical worship of the golden calf. It is worth noting that this idolatrous episode took place at a particular moment when Moses, the moral guiding authority, had left for Mount Sinai to receive the Ten Commandments, the summa of the biblical moral law. But the biblical fall into idolatry took place when a gap had opened between the authority of a father-like figure and the absolute law from above. Could something similar happen with the Parental Alienation, a phenomenon described by Sally Parsloe in her paper?

She brings forth the paradoxes facing the law in divorce cases when the custody of children is involved. First of all the court has to take over the law from the parents who were supposed to represent it for the child. Therefore during a divorce proceedings children are faced with the rule of the law no longer represented and transmitted by the parents. The law outside the family structure will decide, judge and rule on the parents' role over the child; the moral authority of the parents is put on hold. The trauma of divorce may result mainly from this disappearance of the genitorial authority, which appears in turn to be subjected to a higher one, the law of the adults who, like children, must obey, as much as Moses in the face of God. It is exactly in this gap, when the image of the ego-ideal is threatened, that effects similar to idolatry towards the more alienating parent, and soul-murder towards the other parent, take place.

Here we have a facet of the Stockholm Syndrome, to which Parsloe's paper very aptly refers. She describes the status of the child as an object of moral abuse for having been reduced to a pawn for one parent to win against the other. But the most striking similarity with the Stockholm Syndrome is that the victim embraces the cause of the more abusive and powerful parent. If the adult is a 'symptomatic' effect of the social order, the child is the 'symptom' of the family structure, as Lacan suggested. Then he was mostly concerned about the dangerous outcome for children tied up with one parent or when the triangulation fails. They usually become the object of abduction and "have the sole function of revealing the truth of this object".[1]

The paradox a divorce court encounters is that, in wanting to respect the wish of the children, it would be forced to award their legal custody to the parent who abused his/her power over them in order to deviously represent the 'family law' for the child. In the Stockholm Syndrome too the abused aligns with the abuser, the upholder of the arbitrary law of the *primal father* of the horde (Freud, 1913) who has all rights over children, women and chattels. The law (of the state) finds itself dealing with the arbitrary law of the primal father, the idol to be worshipped exactly when the Oedipal myth is failing. Oedipus is the drama where the child has to make a choice between killing the threatening father, and then end up ravaged by guilt, or giving up the mother as object of desire. This is the mythical narrative of the Freudian neurotic child torn by his ambivalence, as Parsloe underlines, while trying some compromises with his conscience.

In a divorce trial children cannot afford a time for doubts and manoeuvres against such a definitive turnover. As for anything else they have to catch what's on offer, a more comfortable life, blackmail, a fake narrative or most probably just letting themselves be the sacrificial enjoyment of Stockholm abductors. The super-ego takes over the ideal-ego.

I wonder whether the exponential growth of incest and paedophilia today could be read within this infantilized human position of our immediate gratification era. The adult, an ex-child after all, who was also a sacrificed idol on the altar of the family cloister, can worship their children's violated bodies and deprive them of their soul, their subjectivity. No surprise then that Parsloe's young Danny desired to die for the British Army. "To lay down your life for your country" is something Ideal, worth dying for, rather than being a sacrificial pawn of his parents' petty war.

Then how are we psychoanalysts, psychotherapists, counsellors responding to a call, however feeble, from these young people caught unarmed in the irresistible arms of a deadly drive at sea? The death drive seems to find its way in when the child's call is not taken notice of, receives no attention or becomes distorted and therefore silenced. Anthony McSherry highlights this in his phenomenological listening inspired by Merleau-Ponty's reflection on giving attention or, I would add, after Heidegger's concept of *Sorge*, a taking care, a listening that implies living attention. McSherry's young man is addressing someone who can hear and see his lack of desire but also his curiosity and his anguish. The opposite of an address is when the child's existence consists in being a receptor, who cannot say yes or no to what is offered, whether in scarcity or wealth, with violence or tenderness. We can think of the autistic child grabbing the mother's hand only as a tool to turn the tap on, both reduced to mute robots. McSherry describes an *imaginary* case of a young man who hardly ever leaves his room, with no work or friends, but entranced by his high tech gadgets. He does gaming with his mates, but they seem to occupy only the position required by the rules of the game. The enjoyment of pre-fabricated games does not involve going out to meet girls, who are "nice sometimes but scary", and trying out new paths and possible new encounters. No love, please! It seems that for this young man there is no public square out there, but a 'wasteland', the image McSherry obtains from him.

"His body was too big for his mind", says the therapist, "He never met his father." Maybe his mind was missing the never met parent, that 'holding still', that 'edge of a riverbank', that constitute the edges of our, however fluid and shaky, kernel of reference, which holds us together. We can understand how cutting your own flesh or injecting it with a substance or making strings rotate in a repetitive way, as autistic children do, are a necessity for finding a centre somewhere, be it the sensation from a self-hurt numb body, the rules of videogames or the immobile centre of a rotating string.

Marie-Christine Laznick,[2] a psychoanalyst who works with early autism, called 'psychic resuscitation' the emergency work she carried out with a little girl who had seriously relapsed into a sort of autistic coma. She felt that if she did not intervene immediately the child's mind would never return. She did this by speaking in a rhythm and tone of voice known as 'motherese' prosody, a kind of pitch and rhythm a mother naturally uses when she is surprised and delighted by the baby's ever novel actions: smiles, grimaces, sounds. If speech reflects genuine surprise and delight, it can have a resuscitating impact on autistic comas of very young children. This makes me think of McShelly's experience of the client seeming to respond to his thoughts and visions as if he could read them from his gestures, his bearing, his thoughts between words and silences. The client must have detected a rhythmic pattern of 'fatherese' that the therapist unwittingly was spelling out. By letting him come forward, the therapist was also letting him swim between his own riverbanks, and by letting him swim away the therapist was left with a sense of grief, probably the grieving that the boy's parents were unable to bear!

That the voice reveals the welcoming (or not) of the child's or the adult's coming forward in unexpected ways, also seems relevant in Onel Brooks' paper. First he poses the question of what is relevant both in a case presentation or a session. What is explicit and easier to interrogate or what is left out of our saying? We could see in McShelly's case that the most important communication took place at the level of the therapist's silent thoughts and wishes. Brooke thinks and feels too, but also speaks, offers hypotheses, at times also gives interpretations, such as the young man's apparent indifference as signalling anger. But Brooke wonders about what it is that really gets the work going. After all, language, which constructs theories and ready-made knowledge, can get in the way like a rock that the therapeutic work has to contend with. It can be felt like a distorting element like a stick in the water, as a form of alienation from some supposed authentic self. It is true that the 'linguistic turn' of the last century, which did not spare phenomenology, placed language on the podium of the masters of the self, and that is why it can be viewed as an obstacle against getting to grips with the 'truer things' regarding our young clients. But we tend to disregard that language, from its early lallations onwards, can also be a call or a response to people and objects we sense as emotionally relevant. The mother's voice with its prosodies and rhythms cannot hide the sensorial/sensual elements of what it is saying.

If Lacan states that language is the 'killing of the thing' or of the original psychic event, we can still hear all the vocal traces of what lays still silent in the net of language. To use Brooke's allegory, fish are caught in the lines and bundled in their holes and knots, in the unconscious side of language, we may say. But paradoxically psychoanalysts do not speak a great deal. Exactly because there is the other side of language, its power of suggestion, words that can be hurled at you like a boulder, words that lose their alignment with meaningful 'things' and, like bricks, participate in the erection of social and cultural monuments. This is the side of language that Brooke terms as intellectualist and would rightly ban from a therapeutic discourse. Still we have to reckon with our own philosophies, as they have been chosen and direct our therapeutic choices as well. In the fishing lines of a session we can find among fish and an old boot also certain words which claim attention, heedfulness. Brooke, the therapist, knows how to listen and reply, but the boy keeps 'disappearing', slips away from the net of language, which falls in the waters of consciousness, of clichés of thought and defensive manoeuvres.

Then something keeps happening: the therapist begins to feel sleepy or confused when the boy 'disappears', wakes up when the reanimated boy starts speaking again and then it is time to stop. Is this not the sequel of the relation between John and his father, a man, whose thoughts are occupied elsewhere while silent with his son, until he makes a prank to wake him up? Here the therapist, by identifying to John's slumberous father, was also acting John's disappearance. Only once they could both set the scene of father's abandonment and John's disappearance could words, those the father did not utter, begin to matter, bring forth questions and responses that could change a crystallized scenario. Then, after another abandonment on the part of the father, John sent a final warning: if you don't get me out of here I'll burn the 'good school' down. Apparently yet another prank, but this time it worked! The father was able *to listen to an act* that was a statement, not a prank, not a repetition of the same, and so could give up the idea of 'the good school' panacea. This case seems to highlight how the symptomatic acting of the young is a way of speaking that fails to address the potential interlocutor and that failure becomes a way of life. All John could express, when faced with the words of the therapist, was his disappearance, his statement of despair and solitude. The burning of the school was John's final act, only after he had warned his deaf father.

If acting takes the place of addressing a call, it also stunts the elaboration of thought so that the calculative autistic feature takes its place. Frances Tustin (Tustin, 1992) a well-known expert on autism, quotes the Danish physicist Niels Bohr when he once rebuked his son with '*You are being logical, you are not thinking*'. Today like never before can we witness how our perfected technological and statistical achievements cannot, autistically, interpret their data nor take the consequent action, just like John's father!

The world is *not-thinking* how to defeat this contemporary plague, the most ancient deadly disease, in the name of Science, which also does not know or cannot think how to defeat a virus. No vision, no capacity to step outside compulsive evidence-based protocols and statistical numbers, even failing to impose the basic use of facemasks, while people are dying by the minute. The economy dictates the numbers ... of the dead, *not-thinking* that the longer we procrastinate the defeat of the virus, the longer the defeat of our economies will last.

Also because of calculative interests we are *not-thinking* of the evident consequences of climate change and want to bend the earth at the cost of abolishing its existence.

Out of all our calculative abilities we *cannot think* or see our all-pervasive racism, which both an imperceptible virus, by killing ill-treated ethnic minorities, and a gone 'viral' video of a black man being murdered by the police as a matter of course, could flush out.

Brooke also expresses concerns about the kind of distancing this pandemic has forced on us. This reminds me of Freud's[3] quote from Schopenhauer about the porcupines that, freezing from the winter cold, "crowded very close together to profit from each other's warmth ... But they soon felt one another's quills, which induced them to separate again". And so on, back and forth "until they had discovered a mean distance at which they could most tolerably exist". In the same mode Italy's locked down people went out on their balconies singing to each other 'Embrace me tighter', which went viral on social media and the news. This may well be the human eternal return that makes it possible to stay away from the quills of human cloisters and then *think up* how to return to desired embraces.

✱✱✱✱✱✱✱✱✱✱✱✱✱✱✱✱✱✱✱✱✱✱✱✱✱✱✱✱

Notes

1. Lacan, J. 1990. *Analysis No. 2, "Notes on the Child"*. Melbourne Centre for Psychoanalytic Research, Deakin Printery, Australia
2. Laznik M. C. 2000: « La voix comme premier objet de la pulsion orale » in La revue Psychanalyse et Enfance du Centre Alfred Binet, Paris.
3. Freud S., (1921) *Group psychology and the Analysis of the Ego*, Vol.XVIII, Hogarth Press, London

Disclosure statement

No potential conflict of interest was reported by the author(s).

References

Freud, S. (1913). *Totem and Taboo* (Vol. 13, Standard ed.). Hogarth Press.

Hall, G., Hivernel, F., & Morgan, S. (2009). *Theory and practice in child psycho-analysis*, (Benvenuto B., chap.9 "La Casa Verde: Speech, listening, welcoming in F. Dolto's work"). Karnac.

Lacan, J. (1990). *Analysis No. 2, "notes on the child"*. Melbourne Centre for Psychoanalytic Research, Deakin Printery.

Owen, C., Farrelly-Quinn, S., (2017). *Further notes on the child*, (Benvenuto B. Chap.4 "Dolto, Klein and Lacan in a polylogue or the Agora effect in the Maison Verte-UK"). Karnac.

Recalcati, M. (2019). *The telemachus complex: Parents and children after the decline of the father*. Polity press.

Tustin, F. (1992) *Autistic states in Children*, Routledge.

How might a therapeutic ethos serve young adults? – A commentary

Richard House

ABSTRACT

This engaging symposium opens up the question of therapeutic work with young adults in a consistently engrossing way that is refreshingly unpredictable and richly diverse. Particularly important is the appropriately extensive space given to the cultural context of therapy in late modernity; the impact and implications of the *Zeitgeist* for working therapeutically with young adults; the contested place of training with this client group; and the demonstration of thoughtful and sensitive clinical work with a client group whose 'emerging-adulthood-in-process' necessitates that therapists do all they can *not to get in the way* of the complex developmental struggles of the troubled young adults who find their way into therapy.

Wie könnte ein therapeutisches Ethos jungen Erwachsenen dienen? - ein Kommentar zum Thema

ABSTRAKT

Dieses engagierte Symposium wirft die Frage der therapeutischen Arbeit mit jungen Erwachsenen auf eine durchweg spannende Art und Weise auf, die erfrischend unvorhersehbar und vielfältig ist. Besonders wichtig ist der entsprechend große Raum, der dem kulturellen Kontext der Therapie in der Spätmoderne eingeräumt wird; die Auswirkungen und Implikationen des Zeitgeistes für die therapeutische Arbeit mit jungen Erwachsenen; der umstrittene Ausbildungsort mit dieser Kundengruppe; und die Demonstration einer nachdenklichen und sensiblen klinischen Arbeit mit einer Klientengruppe, deren „aufstrebendes Erwachsenenalter im Prozess" erfordert, dass Therapeuten alles tun, um den komplexen Entwicklungskämpfen der jungen Erwachsenen in Schwierigkeiten, die ihren Weg finden, nicht im Wege zu stehen in die Therapie

¿Cómo podría un ethos terapéutico servir a los adultos jóvenes? – un comentario sobre la cuestión temática

RESUMEN
Este atractivo simposio abre la cuestión del trabajo terapéutico con los adultos jóvenes de una manera consistentemente fascinante que es refrescantemente impredecible y muy diversa. Particularmente importante es el espacio apropiadamente amplio que se da al contexto cultural de la terapia en la modernidad tardía; el impacto y las implicaciones del Zeitgeist para trabajar terapéuticamente con adultos jóvenes; el lugar de formación disputado con este grupo de clientes; y la demostración de un trabajo clínico reflexivo y sensible con un grupo de clientes cuya 'adultez emergente en proceso' requiere que los terapeutas hagan todo lo posible para no interponerse en las complejas luchas de desarrollo de los adultos jóvenes con problemas que encuentran su camino en terapia.

In che modo un *ethos terapeutico* può servire i giovani adulti? - un commento sulla questione tematica

Questo coinvolgente simposio si focalizza sul lavoro terapeutico con i giovani adulti in un modo costantemente avvincente, imprevedibilmente inatteso e riccamente diversificato. Di particolare importanza è lo spazio esteso dato al contesto culturale della terapia nella tarda modernità, l'impatto e le implicazioni dello Zeitgeist nel lavorare terapeuticamente con i giovani adulti, il luogo contestato di formazione con questo gruppo di clienti;e la dimostrazione di un lavoro clinico attento e sensibile con un gruppo di clienti il cui 'processo di maturità emergente' richiede che i terapisti facciano tutto il possibile per non ostacolare le complesse lotte evolutive dei giovani adulti in difficoltà che trovano la loro strada in terapia.

En quoi une philosophie thérapeutique peut-elle servir les jeunes adultes? Un commentaire sur le thème de cette édition spéciale

Avec une imprévisibilité rafraîchissante et des points de vue très divers, ce colloque très intéressant déploie la question du travail thérapeutique avec de jeunes adultes de manière constamment captivante. Ce qui est particulièrement important c'est la place faite au contexte culturel de la thérapie dans la modernité tardive; l'impact et les implications de l'air du temps pour le travail thérapeutique avec les jeunes adultes; la place disputée de la formation avec cette population; et la démonstration d'un travail clinique prévenant et délicat auprès d'une population dont « l'âge adulte-en-devenir » nécessite que les thérapeutes fassent tout ce qu'ils peuvent pour ne pas *se mettre en travers* des épreuves développementales complexes auxquelles font face les jeunes adultes en difficulté et qui trouvent leur chemin dans la thérapie.

Πώς μπορεί να εξυπηρετήσει τους νέους το θεραπευτικό ήθος; - σχολιασμός στις θεματικές του ζητήματος

ΠΕΡΊΛΗΨΗ

Αυτό το ελκυστικό συμπόσιο ανοίγει το ζήτημα της θεραπευτικής εργασίας με τους νέους ενήλικες, με έναν συνεκτικά συναρπαστικό τρόπο, ο οποίος είναι αναζωογονητικά απρόβλεπτος και πλούσιος. Ιδιαίτερα σημαντικά είναι ο κατάλληλα εκτεταμένος χώρος που δίνεται στο πολιτισμικό πλαίσιο της θεραπείας στα τέλη του νεωτερισμού, το αντίκτυπο και οι συνέπειες του Zeitgeist *(πνεύμα των καιρών)* στη θεραπευτική συνεργασία με νεαρούς ενήλικες, οι προκλήσεις στον εκπαιδευτικό χώρο με αυτήν την ηλικιακή ομάδα, και η ένδειξη στοχαστικής και ευαίσθητης κλινικής εργασίας με αυτήν την ομάδα πελατών, της οποίας η «αναδυόμενη διαδικασία ενηλικίωσης» απαιτεί από τους θεραπευτές να κάνουν ότι μπορούν έτσι ώστε *να μην σταθούν εμπόδιο στους σύνθετους εξελικτικούς αγώνες των* προβληματισμένων νέων που βρίσκουν το δρόμο τους μέσω της θεραπείας.

SCHLÜSSELWÖRTER Kindheit; Moderne; Technologie; kleine-Erwachsene; Schulsysteme; Therapeutische Erziehung; Klinische Exzellenz; Training; Covid19 Pandemie

PALABRAS CLAVE infancia; modernidad; tecnología; mini-adultos; sistemas de escolarización; educación terapéutica; excelencia clínica; formación; Pandemia de Covid19

MOTS-CLÉS enfance; modernité; technologie; mini-adultes; système scolaire; éducation thérapeutique; excellence clinique; formation; pandémie COVID 19

ΛΈΞΕΙΣ ΚΛΕΙΔΙΆ παιδική ηλικία; νεωτερισμός; τεχνολογία; μικροί ενήλικες; εκπαιδευτικά συστήματα; θεραπευτική εκπαίδευση; κλινική αριστεία; εκπαίδευση; πανδημία Covid19.

What can we recognise of the violence to the young person of the adult world … the impossibility of creating a world where young people are truly protected.

('The narratives of parental alienation')

It is possible to pay attention, to wait, to allow what may come to mind and not turn away …. What seems most important is that we catch ourselves weaving ropes of thought that bind us, and others, and wonder about that.

('Looking back with meaning … ')

We are impoverished and impoverishing if we cling only to what is rational, conscious, clear and well thought out.

('Finishing school, fishing and flourishing')

It is a very welcome, freeing experience to be afforded a canvas on which to scribe one's own commentary on a group of papers that speak directly to one's own interests. I've been thinking and writing about the issues touched upon in this theme issue for over two decades now, very much informed by critiques of the Audit Culture (Power, 1997), humanistic approaches to learning and education (Aloni, 2007) and Steiner Waldorf pedagogy (e.g., Petrash, 2000; Steiner, 1972) – a key moment of which process was the open letter Palmer and I co-organised in 2006 (Palmer & House, 2006), which led to a major conference at the University of Roehampton in 2006 (referred to in the Editorial), another conference and subsequent special theme issue of this journal on play (EJPC (European Journal of Psychotherapy & Counselling), 2008; House, 2008), and then the anthology that Loewenthal and I co-edited in 2009, with its beautiful foreword by Williams (Williams, 2009).

The world today – Britain leaving the European Union, Extinction Rebellion, Covid, 5 G and the technocratic 'march of the inhuman' (Naydler, 2020; Sim, 1999) – looks very different from that which formed the backdrop to our open letter in 2006. I'm therefore more interested in the themes in these papers that deepen, and take to new places, these previous concerns, and in the new questions and problematics to which the changed conjuncture gives rise.

In this commentary, I will refer to the papers under consideration thus: the editorial simply as 'Editorial'; 'The time it takes: how do we understand personal growth in an age of instant solutions?' as 'Time it takes'; ' Training for counselling young people – what is added by a child and adolescent specialism?' as 'Training'; ' The narratives of parental alienation' as 'Parental alienation'; 'Looking back with meaning: an imaginary phenomenology of working with a young adult' as 'Imaginary phenomenology'; and 'Finishing school, fishing and flourishing appetite: engagement and compliance in Daoism, existentialism and psychoanalysis' as 'Finishing school'.

Del Loewenthal's Editorial immediately – and rightly – foregrounds the key question of whether modern society is really bad for young adults. This is a question on which controversy has raged since Palmer's path-breaking book *Toxic Childhood* came out in 2006; and the answer to this question clearly has profound implications for the therapeutic stances and sensibilities that professionals and clinicians take up in relation to their work with young people. For if what I often call 'hyper-modern' technological society (or 'late capitalism') is indeed generating a toxic milieu for young people, then if therapists want to be anything more than sticking-plaster apologists for the status quo, then they are going to have to address these questions – or else something akin to clinical impotency and irrelevance beckon. If they ever did exist, the days of keeping 'the cultural' and 'the political' out of the consulting room are surely over.

In March 2010 I spoke at the Westminster Media Forum conference on 'Children in the commercial world', at which Professor David Buckingham presented his UK government-commissioned report looking at the impact of the commercial world on children's well-being (Department for Children, Schools and Families, 2009; see also Buckingham, 2000). Some rather derogatory references were made at this event about the allegedly 'unscientific' nature of Palmer's work on 'toxic childhood' (Palmer & House, 2006) – as if the question of science and scientific evidence were not themselves highly problematic notions! (e.g., Couvalis, 2013; Feyerabend, 2011). I found it very telling that Palmer was not contacted at all in the researching of this government-commissioned report (Palmer, personal communication). It is very easy to play 'the positivist card' (let's call it) in order to silence turbulent priests who are daring to raise fundamental questions about the currently prevailing *Zeitgeist*; and the history of the sciences is replete with such highly dubious moves underpinned by the ideology of 'normal science' (Kuhn, 1962), as it seeks to assert its hegemony, and silence all opposition.

Buckingham's report states, for example, that 'The validity of these [toxic childhood] arguments ... rest[s] on a series of broad assertions about the changing nature of childhood and family life that are in many cases highly debatable' (Department for Children, Schools and Families, 2009, p. 28). Yet we are not told in what ways they are debatable, and how, methodologically, one might go about producing 'evidence' that is not 'debatable'. Certainly, in a critically informed, 'post-positivistic' approach to research, the kind of wide-ranging and complex discursive evidence produced by Palmer can be seen as making a very important contribution, which a more positivistic approach – narrowly focusing on that which is easily measurable, and then assuming that those data adequately capture the full story – is less capable of providing. And recent work by Creasy and Corby (2019) adds strong corroboration to Palmer and others' concerns about the relentless denuding of childhood experience.

In 'Time it takes', we read of 'the consumerising of human experience', with 'more and more aspects of our lives ... being reduced, explicitly or implicitly, to the level of commodities' – with human rights now treated as possessions, and 'a whole range of relationships ... being reimagined in these terms of producer and consumer'. The author is surely right in saying that we need to start thinking deeply about, 'and identify some of the areas in our culture that play into, the commodifying mentality'; and 'the commodified world of late modernity' needs to be resisted, 'with its impatience and its love-affairs with instantaneous solutions and gratifications'.

We might even refer here to *the neoliberal colonisation of the human psyche* (see, for example, Verhaeghe, 2014). Thus, we see the modern, alienating 'pay-for-performance mentality', with its imperative to achieve and be happy, and which is arguably generating a warped view of the self, major disorientation and even despair, with people lonelier than ever before, and love often absent as young people struggle to find meaning in their lives. Three decades of neoliberal free-market ascendancy, rampant privatisation, and the impact of our 'engineered' society on personal identity surely have much to answer for. Nearly two decades before Verhaeghe, Sloan was poignantly asking, 'Could it be that societal modernization is linked to increased emotional suffering on a broad scale? ... Could one define a set of socio-political strategies that would address effectively the problematic features of modernity?' (Sloan, 1996, p. vii; see also the *Guardian* press Open Letter on the mental health effects of austerity policies in the UK – House & 441 others, 2015a).

In her work on 'toxic childhood', Palmer is also daring to speak of the overwhelmingly materialistic age we live in, and the impact that the materialistic-technological *Zeitgeist* might well be having on children's experience, and on children's development in all kinds of subtle ways that narrow empirical research, which focuses only on what is easily measurable and then assumes that those metrics accurately 'capture' and represent 'reality' (House, 2010, 2019–20), may well not get even close to illuminating in an adequate-enough way. Psychoanalytic theory, for example, can tell us something of children's very subtle developmental process – including, not least, the way in which children learn about desire, and about their own desire. Commercialisation, markets and consumerism are all about desire, and about feeding, and even manipulatively generating, children's materialistic desire.

The commercialisation of childhood experience, and all the attendant technologies, is something that philosophical, psychoanalytic and psychotherapeutic perspectives have much to say about, in terms of what is actually happening to children in their development through this radical 'toxic mix' of the market and consumerism-materialism. For example, perhaps we need to be taking very seriously the kinds of issues raised by neuroscientist Baroness Susan Greenfield in her claim (Greenfield, 2008) that these marketing-driven technologies may well be interfering with the child's developing brain, generating all manner of quite unpredictable consequences for children's identity development. And while Greenfield tends to focus on younger children (e.g., Greenfield, 2018–19), it's clear that – as all good therapists know – if things go wrong at an earlier age, the developmental knock-on impacts are usually considerable. And therapists are also now beginning – not before time – to look into the possible impacts of social media use on young people's well-being (Balick, 2013; Balick & House, 2020; House, 2019).

I've already referred to the 'Time it takes' paper. It was a surprise and a delight for me to read this paper in this theme issue, as it is surely essential that therapy as a practice is paradigmatically located within human culture (and the evolution of human consciousness – e.g., McGilchrist, 2009), rather than implicitly treated as some kind of abstract universal phenomenon with no historical contingency or trajectory. Surely such an understanding of the historical and transitory nature of one's allegiance to therapy is a necessary condition for possessing the genuine modesty that all effective therapists need to have – which will in turn at least make it less likely that our therapy work will be akin to a modernist *acting-out within the prevailing paradigm* that cannot but uncritically reproduce and reinforce it. Cushman's work, for example, is an excellent example of someone who believes that locating therapy historically within evolving human culture is an indispensable prerequisite to deeply and reflexively understanding therapy as a practice (Cushman, 1992, 1995).

'Time it takes' helpfully points out that in late modernity, 'the ideal is wakefulness', and that we are infected by 'an undying vigilance around our performance and our control of the environment' – a fantasy, by the way, that I was delighted to see the case material in 'Parental alienation', 'Imaginary phenomenology' and 'Finishing school' radically problematising and deconstructing. The paper's foregrounding of the notion of *rhythm* and its central importance to human health at every level is also most welcome (cf. House, 2004–2005); and natural human rhythms are, of course, one of the first casualties of a hypermodern, control-oriented egotistical culture that uncritically embraces (communication) technologies as some kind of harmless, neutral accoutrement, rather than a technocratic intrusion that, at worst, may well threaten our very humanity (Naydler, 2020; Perlas, 2018; Sim, 1999).

I have long believed that there are rich possibilities in bringing together Merleau-Ponty (Felder & Robbins, 2011) and Rudolf Steiner on these issues. Certainly, young persons' energies can easily be stretched beyond manageable limits if they have to devote undue energy to trying to maintain balance in situations that lack the life and body rhythms that 'Time it takes' refers to. This paper also rightly points out how algorithms 'simply calculate regularities in moments of choice, not the processes of learning to choose' – just one of the many ways of illustrating why the machine can never replicate what is uniquely human (cf. House, 2019–20). All in all, there is a deeply humanistic vision in 'Time it takes that I strongly connected with.

'Time it takes' is also not afraid to point out where therapy alone just isn't sufficient. The author writes, for example:

> If we are concerned to serve and nurture the mental health of a younger generation, we have to look at these broad factors (i.e. the global political, economic and cultural situation we inhabit at present) as well as all the local triggers that generate suffering and confusion for individuals.

In other words, 'therapeutic intervention alone is not the answer … [and] it is all the more important for any therapeutic activity to keep in view these wider questions'. Herein is yet another example of how, paradoxically, the best of therapists will always be radically open to the shortcomings and limits of therapy practice, and the 'politics' that unavoidably accompany it, within a societal context that can never be ignored, underestimated or sidelined.

In short, then, we are faced with 'the loss of a standard narrative of human development'; and this paper's searching question, 'do we have stories about how we have learned to be human?', seems to me to be one that all practising therapists could be very gainfully contemplating throughout their working lives – and of course 'taking their time' to do so!

The other excellent papers in this theme issue should be seen against the backdrop of the preceding discussion, and deserve much more space and attention than I am able to give them here. 'Training' makes a strong and convincing case as to 'why and how a training in child and adolescent counselling offers key insights and skills which help in working with this age group' (a similar case is made by Riha, 2011). On this view, 'emerging adulthood' is *a phase in its own right*, 'which is neither adolescence nor adulthood', and 'their maturational journey remain[ing] very much in progress'. Thinking psychoanalytically, and avoiding undue adherence to a normative developmentalist ideology (Burman, 2007; Morss, 1996), the complexity of the journey into adulthood quickly becomes apparent – and will be even more complex and challenging when a phenomenon like 'Parental alienation' is present. To take just one obvious example, with ever-more children remaining in the family home well into adulthood, 'the emotional difficulty of establishing oneself as an independent individual [being] compounded by the external reality of still being part of the original family at a practical level' is surely going to become an increasingly recurrent developmental vicissitude for this client group.

I also appreciated this paper's engagement with the crucial *psychodynamics* of learning (e.g., Davou, 2002; Mayes, 2009) – one of Freud's celebrated 'impossible professions', of course – and especially relevant here, as a substantial proportion of the 18–24 age group will be in full-time education. Power, group and organisational dynamics are also well covered – though the paper's customary hat-tip to neuroscience is, I must confess, one that I can never really understand the relevance of (House, 2013b). I also found this paper refreshingly non-partisan and lacking in the turf-colonising power-moves that can so often bedevil professionalised therapy.

The three clinical papers – 'Parental alienation', 'Imaginary phenomenology' and 'Finishing school' – were a delight to read; and I hope I'm right in recognising in these papers the rich tradition of Roehampton's Research Centre for Therapeutic Education's approach to therapy – that is, for example, allowing thoughts to come to mind, embracing impossibility and celebrating paradox, staying with 'not-knowing', letting go of firm beliefs and ideas, playing, avoiding over-rationalisation, 'just noticing' rather than interpreting and categorising, getting out of the way, bewaring of calculative knowledge, staying with living thoughts as they arise, noticing what is elided or left out, following faithfully rather than imposing and controlling, abandoning oneself to the call of the moment ... – and with names like Lyotard, Levinas, Heidegger, Husserl, Lacan, Nietzsche, Phillips and, of course, Freud informing the therapists' sensibility to the work.

In therapy work of this nature, moreover, it will sometimes be necessary to articulate, name, and *stay with* the sheer impossibility of the situations clients are in – or 'the impossibility of coming to a clear answer' ('Parental alienation' paper) – thus challenging the 'problem-solving' modernist assumption that there must exist a rational (re)solution to any conceivable circumstance. 'Can we as adults bear to say, "I am sorry. I am not sure I can make it better, but I hear how painful it is and I will listen"' ('Parental alienation').

There is something so freeing and enabling about this approach to therapy (or an 'approach-*which-is-not-one*, in postmodern parlance – e.g., House, 1999; Parker, 1999), where the therapist is not setting out to pre-decide what's wrong with the client, to diagnose and 'fix' them; but rather, is maximally opening up a space of developmental possibility which maximises the likelihood of what needs to relationally emerge to happen in the work, and with the therapist doing everything possible to stop their own defences and counter-transference preoccupations getting in the way of the client's process. This is beautiful work to read about – and young adults who manage to find their way into the consulting rooms of such practitioners are fortunate indeed. I am reminded of a wonderful quotation from Fendler which, while critiquing proceduralist approaches to education, is equally applicable to the kind of therapy process illustrated by these writer-practitioners (in the quotation below, I have substituted 'therapy' for 'education' terms):

> Now there is a reversal; the goals and outcomes are being stipulated at the outset, and the procedures are being developed post hoc. The 'nature' of the [client's experience] is stipulated in advance, based on objective criteria .... Because the outcome drives the procedure (rather than vice versa), *there is no longer the theoretical possibility of unexpected results*; there is no longer the theoretical possibility of *becoming unique in the process of becoming* ['treated'] ... In this new system, evaluation of [psychotherapeutic] policy reform is limited to an evaluation of the degree to which any given procedure yields the predetermined results .... (Fendler, 1998: 57, my italics)

I also see this *anti*-approach to therapy practice (if I may so term it) as entirely fitting to the postmodern age of late capitalism – in great contrast to (for example) CBT, which seems to me to be a classic case of a therapy approach which makes little if any attempt to locate *itself* in an historically informed, reflexive way, and which at worst merely reproduces and reinforces the overly rationalist, 'left-brain' mentality of a control-fixated hypermodernity (McGilchrist, 2009) of which the 'Time it takes' paper is so eloquently critical.

Some 20 years ago I wrote a book titled *Therapy beyond Modernity* (House, 2003), which in retrospect was perhaps even more prescient than I realised at the time. In that book, I tried – however inadequately – to set out just why conventional, professionalised therapy is unavoidably a creature (and reinforcer) of modernity; and that if, in the evolution of consciousness, we wish to transcend a woefully unbalanced 'left-brained' modernity (McGilchrist, 2009) and help therapy as a praxis to embrace approaches and ways of being that assist in that process, then radical post-modern, phenomenological and spiritual worldviews offer just some of the avenues we can fruitfully pursue. In this latter sense, I was delighted to read the case material in this theme issue, as these therapist-writers brilliantly illustrate how the best therapy does not jump to diagnostic, theory-driven general-isations, is able to embrace not-knowing and negative capability, and does not need to flee into premature closure to avoid the discomfort of not-knowing, ambiguity and the ineffable.

The theme issue's Editorial presciently raises the question of the possible mental-health impact on young people of the current global pandemic – but at its time of writing, we did not have the information that is available to us now. Just yesterday as I write, a new research report was published showing that young adults in the 18–24 age-range have been disproportionately impacted by 'lockdown' compared with the general population (Mental Health Foundation, 2020, online). Thus, we read that their study consistently found that 'young adults were more likely to report stress arising from the pandemic than the population as a whole. Findings from the third week of June show that 18–24 year olds were still more likely than any other age group to report hopelessness, loneliness, not coping well and suicidal thoughts/feelings'. While it is not clear from the report whether this merely represents a greater *propensity* for young people to report distress rather than a higher incidence of distress per se, there are clearly prima facie concerns that the pandemic has greatly impacted upon young people. In this regard, the MHF continues that 'Young adults have been especially badly hit during the pandemic with a triple whammy of curtailed education, diminished job prospects and reduced social contact with peers'.

In terms of implications, we read further that 'There is an urgent need to put in place special measures to support the mental health and wellbeing of young people age 18–24 with a particular view to addressing uncertainty around employment opportunities and education provision'. So while we keep hearing about the tsunami of mental-health problems that pandemic and lockdown have and will precipitate, it seems clear that the particular mental-health problems of young adults are going to become a central preoccupation of therapists for perhaps some years to come – thus making the timing of this theme issue especially apt. Such therapy work is likely to require highly effective practitioners, working with a client group with already complex presenting issues, which are then further interpenetrated and complexified by the overlay of the pandemic and lockdown, and their manifold effects.

With regard to education, fundamental questions are (thankfully) now being raised about the schooling system itself: for example, is Ofsted (England's controversial schools inspectorate – House, 2020) an institution that we wish to continue in its current role of enforcing the Audit Culture and its narrow view of education? And is the very institution of schooling itself something that needs fundamental re-thinking? (Dusseau, 2020; Glöckler, 2020; House, 2007; Little & Roberts, 2020). Certainly, the pandemic has opened up unexpected possibilities for looking closely at the institutional schooling status quo – and if it is fit for purpose, whether we consider its pre- or post-pandemic nature.

Concluding thoughts

In the UK we insanely criminalise children as young as 10 years of age (see Daw, 2020); we drive young children into formal schooling (House, 2013a) and quasi-formal learning (House, 2015b) at far too young an age; and as pointed out so clearly in 'Time it takes', we insert young children into capitalist relations and hyper-consumerism at far too young an age (House, 2005). Little wonder, then – as Sue Palmer and I warned back in 2006 – that we have an epidemic of mental-health problems.

If all this isn't a paradigm case of the unthoughtfully hyper-rationalist treating of children as 'mini-adults', in the process completely denying the salience of consciousness evolution in human development, I don't know what is. For children's consciousness is fundamentally different from that of adults (House, 2009; Steiner, 1988), and it is a fundamental error – that is, alas, made again and again – that children are not being treated in a way that recognises that their consciousness is qualitatively different from that of adults. This insight strongly supports the argument in the 'Training' paper, that one cannot at all assume that training in adult psychotherapy will sufficiently or adequately equip therapists for making the most effective therapeutic offer to young-adult clients.

I had the pleasure of working in Roehampton University's Research Centre for Therapeutic Education for some seven years – a centre years ahead of its time in that in its very name, it was highlighting the crucial importance of education being a therapeutic (or healing) experience – something that Rudolf Steiner emphasised a century ago, Susan Isaacs picked up on in her wonderful writings on play in the 1930s (e.g., Isaacs, 1933), and which becomes ever-more self-evident as the malaise young people are experiencing in late-modern culture escalates – as the 'Time it takes' paper demonstrates so evocatively. This is actually a centrally *humanistic* view of education (Aloni, 2007), in which those concerns and preoccupations which define our very humanity must take centre stage within any schooling system, with (for example) the ethos of the liberal arts (Fry & Kolb, 1979; Tubbs, 2014) and the perennial virtues (Sardello, 2002) taking precedence over the technological and the Audit Culture graveyard (respectively, House, 2007; Loewenthal, 2009). As 'Time it takes' rightly has it, 'any educational institution that does not make room for the life of faith and the life of imagination is not going to serve the needs of its students or staff in terms of sustainable well-being'.

The casual, unthoughtful treating of children as if they are 'mini-adults' is something being fuelled by diverse forces and interests throughout modern society – interests that have a material stake in children growing up into 'savvy little consumers', from whom money can then be made at younger and younger ages (Beder, 2009). These influences are even now spreading into the kindergarten and nursery, and this is something that surely has to be of major concern – and which of course has major implications for young adults subjected to such regimes, too. Perhaps we need to talk about a *precautionary principle* here – namely, that if there is any doubt at all about children's well-being being compromised by the kind of world that we are creating for them, then a precautionary approach should be informing the very heart of the policy-making process.

I also want to speak here against the kind of unarticulated fatalism that often operates in these conversations about young adulthood in late modernity. I'm referring here to the view that, 'Well, we're stuck with the sort of commercial world we have: that's just progress and the way it is, so we just have to accept and make the best of it. And we certainly can't turn the clock back to some mythical nostalgic past ... ' etc. etc. I see this latter as a fundamentally victimhood-driven viewpoint (Hall, 1993) – the view that we are all somehow victims of modern technology and corporate capitalism, rather than having the will and the capacity to choose different kinds of values and different kinds of lives for our children.

There are many thousands of families out in the world who are actively doing just that – with some having discovered home schooling during lockdown (Dusseau, 2020) – and who, in their own families, are finding ways to live lives which are not dominated by commerce, materialism, media and technology, and who are succeeding in (at the very least) placing in the background the values of consumerism, material desire, communication technologies, and so on. So it's just not true that we are helplessly and hopelessly subject to huge technological processes over which we have no control. We *do* possess the capacity to make informed decisions in these areas of human experience, and to address our human tendency to become addicted to all manner of ephemeral, superficial 'experience-hits' (Postman, 1986) – if only we will consciously exercise the ethical authority and the will for making those healthy and informed choices. And the more responsible adults/parents find the capacity to make such choices, the less fraught young adults' 'emergence into adulthood' is likely to be.

Acknowledgments

I would like to thank the two anonymous reviewers' helpful comments on a first draft of this commentary.

Disclosure statement

No potential conflict of interest was reported by the author(s).

References

Aloni, N. (2007). *Enhancing humanity: The philosophical foundations of humanistic education*. Springer.

Balick, A. (2013). *The psychodynamics of social networking: Connected-up instantaneous culture and the self*. Routledge.

Balick, A., & House, R. (2020). Interview: Psychologists on the case of social networking. *Self & Society: International Journal for Humanistic Psychology, 48*(1), 41–51. https://tinyurl.com/y3ttyg3v

Beder, S. (2009). *This little kiddy went to market: The corporate capture of childhood*. Pluto Press.

Buckingham, D. (2000). *After the death of childhood: Growing up in the age of electronic media*. Cambridge; Polity.

Burman, E. (2007). *Deconstructing developmental psychology* (2nd ed.). Routledge.

Couvalis, G. (2013). Feyerabend, critique of rationality in science. In B. Kaldis (Ed.), *Encyclopedia of philosophy and the social sciences* (pp. 356–360). Sage.

Creasy, R., & Corby, F. (2019). *Taming childhood?: A critical perspective on policy, practice and parenting*. Palgrave Macmillan.

Cushman, P. (1992). Psychotherapy to 1992: A historically situated interpretation. In D. K. Freedheim (Ed.), *History of psychotherapy: A century of change* (pp. 21–64). American Psychological Association.

Cushman, P. (1995). *Constructing the self, constructing America: A cultural history of psychotherapy.* Addison-Wesley.

Davou, B. (2002). Unconscious processes influencing learning. *Psychodynamic Practice, 8*(3), 277–294. https://doi.org/10.1080/1353333021000019024

Daw, C. (2020). *Justice on trial: Radical solutions for a system at breaking point.* Bloomsbury Continuum.

Department for Children, Schools and Families (2009). *The Impact of the Commercial World on Children's Wellbeing: Report of an Independent Assessment.* Prepared by D. Buckingham & others. Dept for Children, Schools and Families and Dept for Culture, Media and Sport. Retrieved 25 July, 2020, from. https://tinyurl.com/y5jsj5qa

Dusseau, A. (2020). *The case for home schooling: A free range education handbook.* Hawthorn Press.

EJPC (European Journal of Psychotherapy & Counselling). (2008). *Special issue on play and playfulness,* R. House & D. Loewenthal. Vol. 10. Taylor and Francis.

Felder, A. J., & Robbins, B. D. (2011). A cultural-existential approach to therapy: Merleau-Ponty's phenomenology of embodiment and its implications for practice. *Theory & Psychology, 21*(3), 355–376. https://doi.org/10.1177/0959354310397570

Fendler, L. (1998). What is it impossible to think? A genealogy of the educated subject. In T. S. Popkewitz & M. Brennan (Eds.), *Foucault's challenge: Discourse, knowledge and power in education* (pp. 39–63). Teachers College Press, Columbia University.

Feyerabend, P. (2011). *The tyranny of science.* Polity Press.

Fry, R., & Kolb, D. (1979). Experiential learning theory and learning experience in liberal arts education. In S. E. Brooks & J. E. Althof (Eds.), *New direction for experiential learning: Enriching the liberal arts through experiential learning* (pp. 79–92). Jossey-Bass.

Glöckler, M. (2020). *Education for the Future.* InterActions.

Greenfield, S. (2008). *ID: The quest for identity in the 21st century.* Sceptre.

Greenfield, S. (2018–19). The use of digital technology and the health and wellbeing of children and young people. *Association for Humanistic Psychology Magazine for Self & Society, 2*(Winter), 4pp. Retrieved 24 July, 2020, from https://tinyurl.com/rj28ter

Hall, J. (1993). *The reluctant adult: An exploration of choice.* Prism Press.

House, R. (1999). Deconstruction, post-?-modernism and the future of psychotherapy (review feature on Ian Parker [ed.], *Deconstructing psychotherapy,* Sage, 1999). *The Psychotherapy Review, 1*(7), 322–332.

House, R. (2003). *Therapy Beyond Modernity: Deconstructing and Transcending Profession-centred Therapy.* Karnac Books.

House, R. (2004–2005). Flowing into healthy development: Cultivating rhythm and repetition in early childhood. *The Mother Magazine, 12*(Winter), 12–14.

House, R. (2005). Born to consume? – Understanding and transcending the materialism rampaging through modern culture. *The Mother Magazine, 15* (Autumn), 34.

House, R. (2007). Schooling, the state and children's psychological well-being: A psychosocial critique. *Journal of Psychosocial Research, 2*(July–Dec), 49–62.

House, R. (2008). Play and playfulness in therapeutic and educational perspectives. *European Journal of Psychotherapy and Counselling, 10*(2), 101–109. https://doi.org/10.1080/13642530802076094

House, R. (2009). The mind object and 'dream consciousness': A Winnicottian and a Steinerean rationale for challenging the premature 'adultisation' of children. In

R. House & D. Loewewnthal (Eds.), *Childhood, well-being and atherapeutic ethos* (pp. 155–169). Karnac Books.

House, R. (2010). 'Psy' research beyond late-modernity: Towards praxis-congruent research. *Psychotherapy and Politics International, 8*(1), 13–20. https://doi.org/10.1002/ppi.204

House, R. (2013a). Approaches to school starting – A global issue. *The Mother Magazine*, 60 (Sept/October).

House, R. (2013b). Letter to the editor: Seductions of neuroscience. *Therapy Today*, (July).

House, R. (2015a). Able, but unready: Accelerated children's learning and development is a toxic phenomenon. *Teach Early Years Magazine, 5*(8), 33. Retrieved 5 September, 2020, from https://tinyurl.com/y5l4fvr9

House, R. (2015b). Letter: Austerity and a malign benefits regime are profoundly damaging mental health. *The Guardian*. 17 April; Retrieved 25 July, 2020, from https://tinyurl.com/k7uaj2m

House, R. (2019). Book review article: The psychodynamics of social networking. *Association for Humanistic Psychology Magazine for Self & Society, 3 Summer*. Retrieved 3 June, 2020, from https://tinyurl.com/y4srnpuc

House, R. (2019–20). Review essay: On the quantification of the social, and its vicissitudes. *Association for Humanistic Psychology Magazine for Self & Society, 4* (*Winter*), 7pp. Retrieved 17 June, 2020, from https://tinyurl.com/y9s8qc3a

House, R. (2020). *Pushing back to Ofsted: Safeguarding and the legitimacy of Ofsted's inspection judgements – A critical case study*. InterActions.

House, R., & Loewenthal, D. (Eds.). (2009). *Childhood, well-being and atherapeutic ethos*. Karnac Books.

Isaacs, S. (1933). *Social development in young children*. Routledge & Kegan Paul.

Kuhn, T. S. (1962). *The structure of scientific revolutions*. Chicago University Press.

Little, G., & Roberts, H. (2020). Build back better: A manifesto for education. *Morning Star*, 11 June; Retrieved 25 July, 2020, from. https://tinyurl.com/yy28vu26

Loewenthal, D. (2009). Childhood, well-being and a therapeutic ethos: A case for therapeutic education. In R. House & D. Loewewnthal (Eds.), *Childhood, well-being and atherapeutic ethos* (pp. 19–35). Karnac Books.

Mayes, C. (2009). The psychoanalytic view of teaching and learning, 1922–2002. *Journal of Curriculum Studies, 41*(4), 539–567. https://doi.org/10.1080/00220270802056674

McGilchrist, I. (2009). *The master and his emissary: The divided brain and the making of the western world*. Yale University Press.

Mental Health Foundation. (2020). *Coronavirus: The divergence of mental health experiences during the pandemic*, 9 July; Retrieved 25 July, 2020, from https://tinyurl.com/y4xe5qo7

Morss, J. R. (1996). *Growing critical: Alternatives to developmental psychology*. Routledge.

Naydler, N. (2020). *The struggle for a human future: 5G, augmented reality and the internet of things*. Forest Row. Temple Lodge Publ.

Palmer, S., & House, R. (2006). Modern life leads to more depression among children (letter). *Daily Telegraph*, 12 September; Retrieved 21 July, 2020, from. https://tinyurl.com/mfcwol

Parker, I. (Ed.). (1999). *Deconstructing Psychotherapy*. Sage.

Perlas, N. (2018). *Humanity's last stand: The challenge of artificial intelligence – A spiritual-scientific response*. Forest Row. Temple Lodge.

Petrash, J. (2000). *Understanding Waldorf education: Teaching from the inside out*. Gryphon Press.

Postman, N. (1986). *Amusing ourselves to death: Public discourse in the age of show business*. Penguin Putnam.

Power, M. (1997). *The audit society: Rituals of verification*. Oxford University Press.

Riha, A. (2011). *Being a professional chameleon: Working with children as a counselling psychologist*. Unpublished Psych.D. thesis, School of Human and Life Sciences, University of Roehampton.

Sardello, R. (2002). *The Power of the soul: Living the twelve virtues*. Hampton Roads Publishing.

Sim, S. (1999). *Lyotard and the Inhuman*. Icon Books.

Sloan, T. (1996). *Life choices: Understanding dilemmas and decisions*. Westview Press.

Steiner, R. (1972). *A modern [new] art of education: Fourteen lectures given in Ilkley, Yorkshire, 5–17 August 1923*. Rudolf Steiner Press.

Steiner, R. (1988). *The child's changing consciousness and Waldorf education*. Anthroposophic Press.

Tubbs, N. (2014). *Philosophy and modern liberal arts education*. Palgrave Macmillan.

Verhaeghe, P. (2014). *What about me? The struggle for identity in a market-based society*. Scribe Publications.

Williams, R. (2009). Foreword. In R. House & D. Loewenthal (Eds.), *Childhood, well-being and a therapeutic ethos* (pp. xv–xviii). Karnac Books.

Young adulthood, well-being and a therapeutic ethos: a case for therapeutic education[1]

Del Loewenthal

It is argued that if therapeutic education is considered as enabling a return to learning from experience, then not only it is important to develop psychological therapies which are not primarily subject to such technological intrusions as our audit culture (Power 1999), but also that far greater consideration should be given to developing societal interventions, such that the need for future psychological therapies is secondary. Whilst the notion of well-being is considered in broad terms, specific reference is made to young adults and children.

However, we first need to consider what it might mean for our society to have an appropriate therapeutic ethos and how we might achieve this. Only then can we consider whether such technological approaches as audit are helpful or detrimental to this purpose. In order to illustrate this, the term 'well-being' is explored and, in particular, how we can provide an enabling, dynamic environment both for our young adults and, through them, for ourselves, which in turn potentially enables us to make a better world. Michael Power in *The Audit Society* (1999) warns us of the audit explosion, which in the UK started in the 1980s with its emphasis on new public management, accountability, transparency and quality assurance. This application to measuring the well-being of our society is loosely based on the notion of financial auditing, which, as an inferential practice, draws conclusions from a limited inspection of documents.

This chapter, in part, critiques audit, and audit culture, with particular reference to Plato's *Therapeia*. Plato suggested that *Therapeia* is of vital importance to our societies. He posited that, whilst scientific and technical knowledge are important, they should always be secondary to the resources of the human soul (Cushman, 2002). Yet, a glance at our educational system with the increasingly central importance given to positivistic auditing, together with the peripheral place of the arts, suggests that we are increasingly in a society where technology comes first, science second and the resources of the human soul a poor third. So, assuming that we want to, how can we change the emphasis so that technology can help develop the potential of our young adults and children? Such tools as audit could return to being seen more as a rule of thumb and not as something that we are systematically governed by. It is as if being subject to audit technology gives some a false sense of control. In contrast, it is argued here that it is sometimes better to be subject to that which we can never fully explain and, by being able to stay with such inabilities, we can be more open to our potency and potentiality. Otherwise, in the deadness of technical 'thinking', we can only be less alive in terms of what some have variously described as a false self (Winnicott, 1965), inauthenticity (Sartre, 1956) or alienation (Marx, 1844/1969).

At the Southern Association for Psychotherapy and Counselling's (SAF-PAC's) Research Unit for Therapeutic Education (RUTE) in the UK, we are particularly interested in exploring the psychological therapies (including psychoanalysis) as enabling a return to learning through experience. Yet, this is so often only once the damage has already been done. If one considers health in terms of primary, secondary and tertiary (World Health Organisation, 2001), then primary health, in respect of the psychological therapies, could be seen as attempting to reduce those aspects of our culture, which harm our souls and don't enhance the development of a culturally facilitative environment. Regarding the distinction between psychotherapy and counselling (which I do not think necessarily has to be made), counselling could be seen as secondary in its attempt to deal with immediate problems and psychotherapy could be seen as being tertiary in reducing the possibility of the problem reoccurring. It is therefore argued here that therapeutic education must be considered, not only in terms of the consulting room, but in terms of influencing our wider culture and thus calling for a greater emphasis on therapeutic education as primary health.

In both the Report of the Children's Society (Layard and Dunn, 2009) and Ecclestone and Hayes' book *The Dangerous Rise of Therapeutic Education* (2008) grave concern is raised, in different ways, about the rise of individualism. For those such as Ecclestone and Hayes, counselling and psychotherapy are very much part of the problem rather than the solution. Whilst agreeing with them that a self-centredness can be reinforced by many therapeutic approaches and that our responsibility to be there for each other can be wrongly taken out of our hands (including the teachers'), it is possible for psychological therapies to encourage a culture that helps us consider others more rather than less. Also, very fortunately, we have Plato's concept of Therapeia, which will be introduced here at length as he was concerned that, without it, we were 'surely destined to disintegrate under the corrosive force of rampant individualism' (Cushman, 2002: 35).

I think it is true that ego psychologists and many behaviourists, existentialists, psychoanalysts and humanists do attempt to create a situation where the client/patient is led to think they are the centre of the world and can have reflected back to them the self-image they think they would like to have (and which most likely never existed). Yet Freud, for one, wrote about our soul, which not by chance Anglo-Americans failed to translate into English (Bettelheim, 1984). Most importantly, he suggested we were subject to our unconscious. It could be argued that Freud and certainly post-Freudians brought in technology in the name of science which subsequent psychological therapists and their patients/clients have been subject to in a different sense and, some would say, to their detriment. Subsequently, with the help of structural linguistics, Lacan added that we are also subject to language, one consequence of which is that words speak us rather than being spoken by us. This perhaps shows more clearly how we are always subject to. Lacan in changing Descartes' 'I think therefore I am' to 'I am where I do not think' can, for one, be seen, in its de-centring, to reopen therapeutic potential, in contrast to a modernistic notion of individualism (Lacan, 2001; Loewenthal and Snell, 2003).

Yet, once again, there is the danger, as can be explained by, for example, Hegel's dialectic that through such an emerging synthesis, another psychological therapeutic technology emerges (in this case 'Lacan-ese') in an attempt to fight what is seen as the current dominant theology. Consequently, this becomes less effective in awakening our souls.

Audits and technological 'thinking' can be fine if they enable us to think, but not if they restrict the essential human basis of our thinking and acting which is what happens when we have an 'audit culture'. Audits can have implications that should not be applied as the basis of our well-being (the same could be said of psychotherapeutic theories). Thus, I think, we can consider the implications of how, as a society, we might remedy our horrendous situation as indicated by UNICEF (2007), where Britain is ranked bottom out of 21 countries in terms of children's well-being. The report highlights how the UK lags on such indicators as the time children spend talking or eating with their parent(s). It seems to suggest that the overall quality of life of the majority of children in the UK and USA is worse than that of much of the rest of the developed world. How has it come about that we could allow such a situation to develop? How is it that as a society we can no longer come to our senses, but have to rely on mechanistic tools such as 'risk management'? Perhaps it is even more the case, as Oscar Wilde said, that we know the price of everything and the value of nothing. It would appear that we no longer know what we value, but is this all part of the way in which we are manipulated through the promise of false securities? To further develop such arguments here, it is as if we vainly hope that there can be external measures – including ones for client and therapist – so that we can ascertain our 'progress' against what is thought of as an external benchmark. Indeed, measures are in place whereby therapists can tell how well they have done after a single session (Jarrett, 2008)!

Before the 1980s, as mentioned, we had rules of thumb but we knew they were just that. Now, in order apparently to help us, we have a positivistic approach, which has fundamentally altered what many regard as research and what we might consider to be our well-being. A number of various technical tools are now used to govern us, rather than to act as indicators, and we are already in what Kierkegaard (1954) would have taken to be the greatest despair, namely the unwillingness to be our own despair.

Perhaps though the unwillingness has also now become an inability, for without a foundation from which to doubt, education through dread is more feared than before.

There are probably many causes of how we have let develop such an audit society, aspects of which can be so detrimental to our children, young adults and ourselves, but how we explore them is vital. For one, as has been mentioned, there is the greater Anglo-American emphasis on a form of empiricism that reinforces modernism. As Cushman (2002), in exploring virtue and knowledge, describes:

> ... in the Sophist ... Plato undertakes to show that crude empiricism is in error since it confuses true reality with that which is not true Being ... It is Plato's intention to show that the Sophist is not talking nonsense but is confounding inferior with superior reality.
>
> (Cushman, 2002: 80)

Can't the same be said about the current strenuous attempt to only consider as evidence that can apparently be empirically measured? Yet such approaches are not inevitable. We saw a different response in France to the cultural challenges of what we know as 'cognitive behavioural therapy' and, in particular, how French psychoanalysis 'seems to be both official and oppositional', enabling the then French Minister of Health to state that 'psychic suffering is neither measurable nor open to evaluation' (Snell, 2008: 276). Such comments from the state then suggest a very different notion of safety from that in the UK.

Another major factor in the potential demise of the quality of children's and young adults' (and our own) lives can be seen as the effect of the Protestant ethic, which has been argued to fuel individualism, perhaps in contrast to many of those continental countries which, though not without their problems, Catholicism has retained a greater influence. (However, here as well, beseeching people to 'love thy neighbour as thyself' can have a downside when it comes to enabling difference!) The need to counter such a Protestant ethic was potentially provided in the twentieth century in terms of the ethics of the relational developed by both Buber and Levinas. Buber (1971) attempted to get us to rethink the other as 'thou' rather than 'it' and through this re-enabled the magic of the relational, which seems so seriously unacknowledged in our educational systems, not least in the training of teachers.

Levinas also emphasised that we are subject-to, for he defined ethics as being subject-to putting the other first (Levinas, 1969). This privileging of heteronomy over autonomy, therefore, would be a far greater influence through a therapeutic ethos both in the consulting room and in our societies. It would counter the very cult of individualism, which the Children's Society and others are so concerned, is ruining the lives of our children and has devastating consequences on the lives of too many young adults.

Here, therefore, we have Jerusalem versus Athens, the book versus the look. So is it possible that schools of education might give a greater emphasis to heteronomous rather than autonomous learners and that chief executives might no longer talk in terms of vision statements in a way that attempts to ensure others are visionless and incorporated? Also, is it possible for psychological therapies not to speak of people as subjects in a way that makes it more likely that others are objects? For, is it possible for two subjects to really meet?

In considering well-being, surely societal and individual perspectives need to be considered. This calls for something other than what we currently understand as the psychological therapies. For example, whilst it is important to consider health as being individually defined (Heaton, 1998), preventative policies are argued here to be vital. In any National Health Service, one doesn't want to put all one's resources into hospitals if one does not have clean water or hygienic sewage systems, and as we seem to be realising, endorsing and encouraging smoking and excessive alcohol consumption and unhealthy eating. Similarly, one doesn't want to put all one's resources into counselling and psychotherapy when one's very education system may be acting against human relationships with our personal behaviour becoming alienated. Perhaps we are now so alienated that we no longer realise that we are experiencing our alienation.

I think Plato's concept of Therapeia is of vital importance when considering such cultural impositions as the place, if any, of audit from the perspectives of both the individual and the state. In attempting to reopen this, I am again particularly grateful for the work of Robert Cushman (2002). From Socrates, therapeutic education can be seen as about awakening thought rather than instilling knowledge. Plato can be regarded as understanding Socrates as the best example of somebody who abounded in the consciousness of well-being, making the soul as good as possible. Furthermore, for Plato, both the ways in which Socrates lived and died were evidence that virtue and well-being are inseparable. For Socrates, the danger is that we are doing the opposite of what we ought to be doing. Rather like today, it is as if good was more to do with the goods we purchase, thus well-being is seen not as primarily about making one's soul as good as possible but rather based upon the 'unexamined supposition' (Cushman, 2002: 13) that good is defined by consumption. Thus, Socrates was against a well-being in terms of 'sensuous satisfactions, together with the largest attainable measure of affluence and personal prerogative' (Cushman, 2002: 13).

For Socrates, the soul is our greatest treasure, so we must first seek virtue. Thus, to Socrates, 'we ought neither to requite wrong with wrong, nor to do evil to anyone, no matter what he may have done to us' (as quoted in Cushman, 2002: 24). In Plato's time, there was already a popular tradition in 'dispraise' of learning. For Plato, it was important for both the individual and the state to give a primacy to seeking wisdom. Plato considered, therefore, that politicians should engender love of virtue and the elimination of injustice in order to make citizens as good as possible. Thus, Plato is pointing out that we can seek the wrong type of education and with it the wrong type of well-being. In order to counter these unhelpful ways of being, Plato further suggests that we cannot rely on religion or the traditions of the elders but of what we must be most wary is the use of rhetoric when it is taught and practised in order to subordinate 'truth to mere persuasiveness' (Cushman, 2002: 36), as practised by Greek spin-doctors, the Sophists, who codified the art of rhetoric, which we have increasingly taken up right the way through to manualised psychotherapies. Yet for Plato, such sophistry always attempts to accommodate itself to the prevailing ethos leaving 'human life unexamined and unchanged' (Cushman, 2002: 36). Importantly, the Sophists, as is so much the case today, 'were not interested in questioning the current fashion of life, only in implementing it' (Cushman, 2002: 36). Eyres (2009) has reminded us, through taking Montaigne (1993) as an example of developing a self-consciousness that may not be about narcissistic individualism, that as with cognitive behavioural therapy this is something that gets applied in the mind rather than within the person.

Interestingly, Plato did not believe that knowledge that constituted virtue was to do with technique, nor did he believe it could be acquired by practice or direct impartation. Knowledge that makes for virtue appears not to be transmissible and therefore cannot be directly taught or obtained through instruction. This then raises the question concerning the nature of the knowledge of those who are virtuous and, if this is obtained by more than just one's nature, what form of learning is entailed. For Plato, 'learning … is something like recovering knowledge out of oneself. This recovery of knowledge under the stimulus of dialectical examination is a case of recollection' (Cushman, 2002: 81). Plato suggests that we go from cognition to re-cognition through a dialectic:

... man, then is a dispossessed possessor of truth about Being. He is half- blind to his own legacy. Although awareness of reality in truth is the mark of his humanity, awareness commonly fails to crystallise and formulate itself into articulate comprehension.

(Cushman, 2002: 84)

For Plato, 'knowledge cannot be put into "a soul that does not possess it" ... Knowledge does not begin with a blank space' (Cushman, 2002: 86). Thus, all cognition is really re-cognition. 'If knowledge, in the last resort, is insight, it manifestly cannot be conveyed even if its condition may be induced' (Cushman, 2002: 88). This implies that conventional notice of instruction had to be replaced by a way 'which would make room for recovery of knowledge out of the self. For such knowledge alone is virtue' (Cushman, 2002: 88).

By means of recollection, true reality begins to be discerned ... [Such] [c]atharsis is more than clarification of the mind to itself. Although [c]atharsis requires the articulation of the presentiments of truth which lie as an unexplored deposit in the human soul, it also involves increase in virtue. Additionally, it is purging of unrighteousness from the soul but [c]atharsis is always something positive, namely replacement of vice by self-restraint, justice, courage and wisdom. Wisdom replaces 'folly' in the soul and is itself the summit of virtue.

(Cushman, 2002: 57)

I am hopeful this very much speaks to, at least, psychotherapists and counsellors. Furthermore, those influenced by psychoanalysis may be interested in further parallels:

Of the two ruling and determining principles in the soul, one leads through intelligence toward what is best. The other is bent upon pleasurable satisfactions. The two are sometimes in agreement within the individual; but with most men, they are in perpetual strife.

(Cushman, 2002: 64)

Therapeutic education therefore needs to be considered, both on a micro and on a macro level. (The micro level might be seen in terms of working with individuals, couples and therapeutic groups.) Therapeutic education does not have to be provided in terms of an individualism where the person can be made to believe that they are like a god returning to situations that in actuality never existed (Borch-Jacobsen, 1989). Anthony Elliott puts the case of how psychoanalysis can possibly correct inappropriate individualism through us being 'subject-to ourselves' (Elliott, 1996). Yet, interestingly Richard Layard talks of the importance of involvement in something greater than yourself (Layard and Dunn, 2009). Here, unlike Layard's insistence on focusing on happiness (Layard, 2006a) and evidence-based psychotherapeutic practice (Layard, 2006b),

I am in agreement with him. For those who are atheist or agnostic and do not see themselves as subject to a god, is it not still possible for them to be subject to such notions as beauty, love, wonderment, spirituality, and the infinite, and to have a therapy which might include some of these considerations, for example, through being subject to an unconscious, language and/or heteronomy? I have previously written about one approach which I termed 'post-existential' but which could enable a search for meaning in a way that we could be subject to such aspects without being caught in a theoretical straitjacket of the wrong sort of knowledge (Loewenthal, 2008a, 2008b).

On a macro level, whilst hopefully the last thing being suggested here is some single policy measure with a rule-of-thumb indicator posing as science, any change perhaps should be seen as an accumulation of many different influences. Nevertheless, as the then Archbishop of Canterbury, Rowan Williams, suggests in his afterword to the report on *A Good Childhood* (Williams, 2009), we do need to consider 'what makes for long-term well-being, otherwise the educating of a new generation is hamstrung from the start'. These macro forces include the emphasis on consumer relations rather than human relations and educational systems, which favour the advantaged over the disadvantaged, ensuring that increasingly our socio-economic systems are generated more by competition than cooperation. As suggested at a recent OECD conference (September, 2007) that I was involved with organising, systems are being developed and encourage greater competitiveness. This is on the assumption that academics do not like teaching and will not like to do the type of research required for tenureship and promotion (OECD, 2007).

We no longer consider what a university might be there for; instead, bland mission statements are issued that seldom seem to consider what a good education might be or what it might mean for a university to be encouraging thoughtfulness, independent yet serving its communities. Such macro developments involve a managerialism, one aspect of which is the development of systems that both encourage individualism and that simultaneously bind the individual as a small cog in a large wheel. It is the choice of these systems that increasingly determine the so-called quality of our lives.

This systematic move away from personal, human relations to market relations can be seen to have influenced our culture in general. For example, in countries such as the UK there has been the demise of trade unions where a history of fighting for our human rights has almost been forgotten and has been replaced by market relations in which the trade union is regarded by members as little more than another service industry. Again, in the UK, the National Health Service no longer considers people to be working together to provide a service by encouraging each other to work for the greater good of humanity through what calls to them. Instead, these attempts to foster the idea of a hospital and hospitality, where we look to welcome a stranger and diminish our own hostile feelings, replacing them with the offer of shelter – traditionally, for some, the breaking and sharing of bread and offering wine – are replaced by competitive systems. These systems of, for example in the UK, 'Foundation hospitals' where people in the same town can be paid different salaries for the same job and where the introduction of such notions as purchasers and providers means that where research is carried out, often with the help of a university. This need not be published if it gives away a local competitive advantage either in terms of showing a good way of doing something or that an existing way is not succeeding as previously hoped. Here, for example, the whole ethos of our university and public health systems has radically changed to encourage a competitive individualism where previous checks and balances such as trade unions, health service professions and academics have been systematically sidelined.

Whilst I would not disagree with those that claim that there did need to be some limits to the power of trade unions, professions and academia when they may have been abusive and not in the 'public interest', the multi-headed movement of managerialism, consumerism and individualism destroyed – and is still destroying – a collective sense, a therapeutic ethos, which is fundamental to the public interest.

There is a prevailing culture whereby universities, through control by central government, are rapidly losing their independence, and public service management is adopting a private model that, again, encourages an individualistic competitiveness over collective action, which is perceived by those in power as a threat rather than enhancing democracy. Indeed, in the UK, the marketing of these changes is such that the reorganised National Health Service is replaced by a series of organisational systems that are given the public misnomer of 'Trusts'.

Another more personal illustration of the demise of everyday human relations is that whilst being brought up in the suburbs of London, I can remember as a family that we knew the name of the cashier of the bank, and when he asked after other members of the family, this was reported at the dinner table. Yet now I'm forever being asked to talk to my unknown 'personal banker' whose name I don't know.

A final example of how, particularly in a UK context, our children and young adults are being brought up in an environment where the assumptions underlying the very language we use to experience being with each other are being systematically changed with regard to 'de-mutualisation'. Mutuals, or Building Societies, are not-for-profit organisations whereby people in the community can save and borrow money at interest rates, which are usually better than a bank that would require profit to pay dividends to their shareholders. Unfortunately, a legal way was found around the mutuality originally intended, whereby for short-term gain the members of a building society could receive a lump sum if their building society was privatised as a bank. One of the consequences of such deregulation was the replacement of competition through a mixed economy (Public, Private and Mutual/Co-operative) with a banking system that subsequently went bankrupt to the profit of a few and the long-term detriment of the majority. However, what we can see from banking in other countries in continental Europe is that whilst there are large, global, cultural shifts, it is possible to have some agency in our responses to them and it is not inevitable that we have to destroy so much of what are good aspects of our heritage that we have painstakingly built up to enable how we are with each other.

Therapeutic education through counselling and psychotherapy can therefore take on the values of individualism and autonomy, but this is not inevitable. It can, for example, give a primacy to heteronomy whilst not ignoring issues of autonomy. However, therapeutic education can also be seen as an additional way of taking responsibility for considering how the therapeutic ethos is affected through economic, social, political and technological changes.

'Well-being' is another term in the title of this chapter. Here I find useful Heidegger's notion of Dasein 'being-in-the-world with others'. Yet again, the way our society is developing is to ensure that there is less opportunity to dwell on what we might mean by well-being. Not untypically, when I asked some researchers presenting at a recent Economic and Social Research Council (ESRC) conference how they defined well-being, I was told they no longer focused on this, but, instead, on how it might be measured. Indeed, increasingly, my experiences of academia are what was previously a standard conceptual exploration is now often dismissed as philosophy and that the philosophy department has often been closed down. Similarly psychology, particularly in the UK and USA which, as previously mentioned, do so poorly in international comparisons of childhood, focuses again on the empirical, forgetting that one of its key founders, Wilhelm Wundt (1904), suggested that the key task of psychology was to marry the empirical with cultural and historical. Similarly, education can be seen as increasingly caught up with pseudo-quantification of aspects of quality that are often in danger of bringing about an ethos which may be more detrimental than beneficial.

Social anthropology, because of the influence of multiculturalism and the relative demise of sociology, together with the study of literature, perhaps provides some of the few remaining places where relationships can be thought about in a social context (though positivism appears to be also creeping in here). Certainly, programmes in counselling and psychotherapy rarely seem to provide a significant critique of their own gurus, let alone considering individual therapeutic interventions within a broader socio-economic context (and attempts to set up, for example, 'Psychotherapists and Counsellors for Social Responsibility' (Samuels, 2003) have not, as yet, entered mainstream thinking). It is even rarer for any university course to consider what impact policy changes might have on how we experience each other. Our higher education system, therefore, is not strong enough to allow the socio-economical questioning of the government who fund most of it, and it could be seen that the ideological control is such that we cannot allow thought to come to us, not only in terms, for example, of a Freudian unconscious, but also in terms of Marxist alienation. It's as if the fall of the Iron Curtain and the knowledge of the horrors of communist totalitarianism have undermined other notions of working together for the common good. We therefore do not see the potential damage we are doing in establishing, perhaps, a more subtle ideological totalitarianism where knowledge is seen in terms of competencies which can always be explicit and measured, and Polyani's notion of tacit knowledge recedes even further (Polyani, 1966).

Perhaps it is the relationship that is the greatest educator of them all. Yet in some ways will it always be mysterious? Here something rather than just being taught and learned is imparted and acquired and might well be a key aspect of how psychotherapy and counselling work (should we ever find out!). It is perhaps important to remember here what Merleau-Ponty warns that sometimes if we try to take away what is mysterious, we end up taking away the very thing itself (Merleau-Ponty, 1945/1956: 70).

Speaking of relationship finally brings me to a further term in the title of this chapter, 'Young adulthood'. It is suggested here that the relationship between the young adult and the adult, as with the child and the adult, is not only of vital importance to the young adult but also to the adult.

Bernstein Miller and Lane (1991) conclude from their study of undergraduates that the results of their research 'are consistent with previous findings that individuation and well-being in adolescence are facilitated by close, positive relationships with parents rather than distancing one's'. Yet what we know of parent and child relationships too often do not provide a foundation for such 'close, positive relationships'.

Instead, what we find are conditions developing which produce a dramatic reduction in the time spent together by adults and children. Parents in the UK spend less time with their children than most other Western societies, despite the fact that all Western societies have technological changes such as central heating, enabling more individual members of families to be in their own rooms with personal TVs, video games, etc. There is also, in the UK, the shocking statistic of how very few male teachers now work in primary schools. It is this last statistic that may provide a clue about how the changing therapeutic ethos leads to an impoverished sense of well-being for our children and ourselves.

Deregulation has also taken part in the more complicated area of censorship. I rarely watch television but I have heard a Friday evening prime-time chat show host saying 'I'm going home for a family wank (whatever that is)', and on another programme I have heard young adults being asked in what ways they thought their parents enjoyed sex best. Their parents then gave, in turn, the 'true answer' etc. Once again, sex is made explicit and measurable but it, perhaps, leaves us to being even less thoughtful and more frightened of ourselves. It's not only male teachers who are frightened of being paedophiles, but in an overtly and increasingly sexually explicit world, parents cannot so easily play with their children or spend time with them, perhaps with the fear that the thoughts that may come to them cannot be shared with anyone.

Through Plato can be seen the importance of play and how the child can uniquely develop through it. Both children and adults need to be able to be trusted and trust themselves to play with each other through being subject to play. We need both to allow time for each other and not let unspeakable anxieties get in the way. The danger is that we become less thoughtful as we become less able to learn through the relational and play. One detrimental effect of this is that we become less playful, not only with each other but with ideas: for example, our preoccupation with increasingly narrow notions of evidence, where it is almost as if we try and believe that if it can't be measured it doesn't exist. Science, and particularly technology, increasingly rules our lives and, in so doing, we become less thoughtful of such developments. Many children and young adults, through the psychological therapies, are able to return to becoming more playful and, hence, more alive, but could more be done preventatively? It is not only people who have been sexually, physically and particularly verbally abused who may find it difficult to learn in an ordinary healthy way through play but, because of increasing cultural concerns such as 'stranger danger' in an increasingly sexualised world, we are becoming a more frozen society and unable to play with our children who, in turn, may become less playful in their own and our lives. Importantly, House (2008) argues how 'the attitudes and way of being to which the "audit culture" inevitably gives rise are … incompatible with those subtle yet essential "play-full" qualities that are the very lifeblood of children's early experience' (House, 2008: 16). Furthermore, Mayo and Nairn (2009) warn us that child's play has become manipulated through the consumer culture leading to children whose resulting materialistic output is, they suggest, correlated with lower self-esteem. This is in contrast to free play, where children can let play emerge with other children. However, whilst our audit culture is potentially robbing us and our children, it would be wrong to end without also taking Fletcher's work (2008) on growing up in England between 1600 and 1914 with its high infant and child mortality and tough social conditions for the majority, to warn us not to be too nostalgic about the past.

In summary therefore, whilst exploring what makes a good counsellor or psychotherapist for a young adult is significant, such considerations of our practice, in terms of the good, may well be healthy but it is suggested in this chapter that therapeutic education is a necessity, not only on an individual level but, more importantly, on a societal one. (Further, this is true not just for young adults but for us all.) If this, for some, does smack of social engineering then it has been argued here that this can still be open to the wonderments of an unknown. Notions of transforming our potential hostility to the stranger into hospitality cannot be left solely to professional therapists. As a profession we will surely fall short unless such notions of 'meeting' are more a part of our culture. This is perhaps more akin to what Plato termed Therapeia.

The growing trend of audit culture with its many managerialist derivatives includes a narrower reading of evidence-based practice, which in turn is significantly changing the provision of therapies. This apparent acceptance of technology, let alone science over wisdom, has significant consequences for the quality of our lives. If we are to be in with a chance of leading a good life, it is essential for therapists to consider how they can influence education in general. Plato intended that if we are to avoid the disastrous consequences arising from the distortion of our souls, then virtue must be a precondition of knowledge.

To Plato, the highest form of knowledge was wisdom, and education is required to revolutionise the mind. Therapeia is therefore the therapy of the soul, and Plato regarded a conversion to be necessary in order to tackle the ignorance of corrupt minds. As psychological therapists, we need to look at therapy as an educational practice, not only as part of what is now increasingly termed 'continuous professional development', or possibly in the consulting room, but in terms of educating our societies to see the wisdom of locating scientific, technical thinking as secondary to the resources of the human soul. For Plato, as for Socrates beforehand, a key question was 'can virtue be taught?'

Cushman (whose book Therapeia is now, sadly, out of print) details available that Plato thought his educational schema was only barely a sufficient antidote to cope with our desperate human plight. For Socrates, the aim of teaching (and this may be familiar for some psychological therapists) was not that it was possible to impart truth, but what others could be led to apprehend as their own discovery. Therefore, such a therapy can be seen not as about knowledge but instead about awakening thought. Plato thus saw Socrates, as some of us might see current psychological therapies, as a physician of souls by means of dialogue.

All this raises a number of questions: perhaps most importantly, can we put the resources of the human soul first so that audits and empirical research become its servant rather than the other way around? Should a psychological therapist's responsibility be to make each soul as good as possible or would this be too much of an agenda? Do we not in some way always imbue our clients/patients with our own value systems? Is therapy about resolving into virtue 'the warfare between the conflicting impulses of the soul'? What if therapy only seems to do this, where 'word juggling' may inappropriately transmute irresponsibility into integrity?

Building on the work of Gadamer (1975), therapy with individuals could be seen as a way of enabling an interrupted process of education, facilitating the return to learning from experience, but this can only really take place, and consequently be sustained, in a society where learning from experience is for the good. We might then examine more healthily what part those in such professions as management and education should undertake with re-gard to those souls for which they have a responsibility (without reducing this to either a manualised set of counselling skills or the non sequitur of 'an ethical code' as if either could be a basis of training), regardless of whether this includes formal psychotherapy/counselling.

Then we could consider more the training of 'good' teachers, supervi-sors and researchers of counselling and psychotherapy in a different way. However, in the first instance, we need as psychological therapists to do everything we can to educate our society concerning questions about the 'good', otherwise we will be at best marginalised, and at worst part of the 'bad'. To return to Therapeia: if we allow Plato to speak, he will suggest that the question before us is whether we shall shrivel on the positivistic vine, or with him, plumb again the resources of the human soul and so recover ....
(Cushman, 2002: xvi)

Note

1 This chapter is developed from Loewenthal, D (2009) *Childhood, wellbeing and a therapeutic ethos*: A case for therapeutic education (Ch 2). In R House and D Loewenthal, Childhood, Wellbeing and a Therapeutic Ethos. London: Karnac Books and Loewenthal, D 2010, Audit, audit culture and therapeia: Some impli-cations for wellbeing with particular reference to children (Ch 6). In L King and C Moutsou (eds), *Rethinking Audit Cultures: A Critical Look at Evidence-Based Practice in Psychotherapy and Beyond*. Monmouth: PCCS Books.

References

Beinstein Miller, J and Lane, M (1991). Relations between young adults and their parents. *Journal of Adolescence*, 14(2), 179–194.

Bettelheim, B (1984). *Freud and Man's Soul*. New York: Random House.

Borch-Jacobsen, M (1989). *The Freudian Subject*. Stamford, CT: Stamford University Press.

Buber, M (1971). *I and Thou*. New York: Free Press.

Cushman, P (2002). *Therapeia: Plato's Conception of Philosophy*. New Brunswick, NJ/London: Transaction Publishers.

Ecclestone, K and Hayes, D (2008). *The Dangerous Rise of Therapeutic Education*. London: Routledge.

Elliott, A (1996). *Subject to Ourselves: Social Theory, Psychoanalysis and Postmodernity*. Cambridge: Polity Press.

Eyres, H (2009). Within you, without you. *The Financial Times*, 11/12 July, p. 20 (Life and Arts).

Fletcher, A (2008). *Growing Up in England: The Experience of Childhood 1600–1914*. Yale, CT: Yale University Press.

Gadamer, H-G (1975). *Truth and Method*. New York: Seabury Press.

Heaton, J (1998). The enigma of health. *European Journal of Psychotherapy and Counselling*, 1(1), 33–42.

House, R (2008). Audit culture and play. *Early Years Educator*, 9(10), 16–18.

Jarrett, C (2008). When therapy causes harm. *Psychologist*, 21(1), 10–12.

Kierkegaard, S (1954). *Fear and Trembling*. New York: Doubleday.

Lacan, J (2001) *Ecrits*. London: Routledge.

Layard, R (2006a). *The Happiness Report: Lessons from a New Science*. London: Penguin.

Layard, R (2006b, June). *The Depression Report: A New Deal for Depression and Anxiety Disorders*. The Centre for Economic Performance's Mental Health Policy Group.

Layard, R and Dunn, J (2009). *A Good Childhood: Searching for Values in a Competitive Age*. London: Penguin.

Levinas, E (1969). *Totality and Infinity*. Pittsburgh, PA: Duquesne University Press.

Loewenthal, D (2008a). Introducing post-existentialism: An approach to well-being in the 21st century. *Philosophical Practice*, 3(3), 316–321.

Loewenthal, D (2008b). Post-existentialism as a reaction to CBT? In R House and D Loewenthal (Eds), *Against and For CBT: Towards a Constructive Dialogue* (pp 146–155). Ross-on-Wye: PCCS Books.

Loewenthal, D and Snell, R (2003). *Postmodernism for Psychotherapists*. London: Sage.

Marx, K (1969). *Economic and Philosophical Manuscripts of 1844*. California: International Publishers. (Original work published 1844)

Mayo, E and Nairn, A (2009). *Consumer Kids: How Big Business Is Grooming Our Children for Profit*. London: Constable.

Merleau-Ponty, M (1956). *Phenomenology of Perception*. London: Routledge. (Original work published 1945)

Montaigne, M (1993). *The Complete Essays* (MA Screech, trans). London/New York: Penguin.

OECD (2007). *Supporting Success and Productivity: Practical Tools for Making your University a Great Place to Work*. London: OECD Directorate for Education.

Polyani, M (1966). *The Tacit Dimension*. New York: Doubleday.

Power, M (1999). *The Audit Society: Rituals of Verification*. Oxford: Oxford University Press.

Samuels, A (2003). Psychotherapists and counsellors for social responsibility (UK). *Journal for the Psychoanalysis of Culture and Society*, 8(1), 150–153.

Sartre, J-P (1956). *Being and Nothingness: An Essay on Phenomenological Ontology*, (H.E. Barnes, trans). New York: Philosophical Library.

Snell, R (2008). L'anti livre noir de la psychoanalyse: CBT in French/Lacanian perspective. In R House and D Loewenthal (Eds), *Against and For CBT: Towards a Constructive Dialogue*. Ross-on-Wye: PCCS Books.

United Nations International Children's Emergency Fund (UNICEF) (2007). *Report on Children in Industrialized Countries*. New York: UNICEF.

Williams, R (2009). Afterword. In R Layard and J Dunn (Eds), *A Good Childhood: Searching for Values in a Competitive Age* (pp 167–178). London: Penguin.

Winnicott, DW (1965). *Ego Distortion in Terms of True and False Self. In The Maturational Processes and the Facilitating Environment*. London: Hogarth Press.

World Health Organisation (2001). *Mental Health: New Understanding, New Hope (The Health Report 2001)*. Geneva: World Health Organisation.

Wundt, W (1904). *Principles of Physiological Psychology* (B Titchener, trans). Cambridge, MA: Harvard University Press.

Index